Integrating Expressive Arts and Play Therapy With Children and Adolescents

Integrating Expressive Arts and Play Therapy With Children and Adolescents

Edited by

Eric J. Green
Athena A. Drewes

WILEY

Cover Design: Andrew Liefer
Cover Image: Kriss Russell/iStockphoto.com

Published by John Wiley & Sons, Inc., Hoboken, New Jersey.
Published simultaneously in Canada.

For general information on our other products and services please contact our Customer Care Department within the United States at (800) 762-2974, outside the United States at (317) 572-3993 or fax (317) 572-4002.

Wiley publishes in a variety of print and electronic formats and by print-on-demand. Some material included with standard print versions of this book may not be included in e-books or in print-on-demand. If this book refers to media such as a CD or DVD that is not included in the version you purchased, you may download this material at http://booksupport.wiley.com. For more information about Wiley products, visit www.wiley.com.

Library of Congress Cataloging-in-Publication Data

Integrating expressive arts and play therapy with children and adolescents / [edited by] Eric J. Green and Athena A. Drewes.
    1 online resource.
    Includes bibliographical references and index.
    Description based on print version record and CIP data provided by publisher; resource not viewed.
    ISBN 978-1-118-77544-8 (ebk) — ISBN 978-1-118-77561-5 (ebk) —
    ISBN 978-1-118-52798-6 (pbk)
        1. Arts—Therapeutic use.   2. Play therapy.   3. Performing arts—Therapeutic use.
    4. Psychotherapy—Practice.   I. Green, Eric J., editor of compilation.   II. Drewes, Athena A., 1948– editor of compilation.
    RC489.A72
    616.89'1653—dc23
                                                                                    2013023348

Printed in the United States of America
10 9 8 7 6 5 4 3 2 1

Eric J. Green

To my young nieces, nephews, and godchildren:
Maddy, Lily, Isabel, Oscar, Katelyn, London, Levi,
Cameron, & Zach. Thank you for teaching Uncle
Eric the true and amazing power of play. I love you!

Athena A. Drewes

To my sons, Scott Richard Bridges and Seth Andrew
Bridges, from whom I draw inspiration and love that sustains
me through all that I do! You are my pride and joy!

Contents

Preface

Welcome to *Integrating Expressive Arts and Play Therapy With Children and Adolescents*. The premise of this book began as an idea in October 2010 at the Association for Play Therapy's Annual Conference in Sacramento, California. Rachel Livsey, Senior Editor at John Wiley, approached me (Green) with an idea. She inquired about my interest in compiling a resource-type book integrating the expressive arts and play therapy frameworks so that clinicians would have ease of access to the ethical considerations and competency implications when developing a multimodal treatment stance.

Little has been written in the literature regarding clinicians seeking to competently integrate the expressive arts into their child play psychotherapy practice. At first, I was ecstatic about the idea. This could be another opportunity for our disciplines to bridge commonalties under the expressive art therapy umbrella, as opposed to us looking at the negatives and the deficits in each other and our training. Sometimes we engage in anxiety-driven, petty turf wars, where unchallenged ideology and rigid doctrine blinds us to the real mission of why we're here in the first place. At this point, I also instinctively knew this project was going to have a bit of a synergistic element, and so it began. First, I implored Athena Drewes to co-edit the volume with me. We sought out the consult of one of the gurus in the expressive arts field, Barry Cohen, who hosts the annual Expressive Arts Therapy Summit in New York City. This summit is a conference where therapists from all of the expressive arts disciplines from all over the world come together to provide trainings from their respective fields of expertise. This is when the book began to take its shape, focus, and soul.

This guidebook's overall premise is meant as a practical illustration for child-based mental health clinicians to competently integrate interventions and approaches from the expressive arts and play therapy disciplines. Moreover, we compiled this volume so that clinicians and graduate students in mental health programs can augment their therapeutic toolkit and training within a competent, research-based practice. The second aim of the book is to provide a resource guide and practical textbook for educators in university settings who teach either play therapy or one of the disciplines in the expressive arts that seek to integrate disciplines for holistic care of children, adolescents, and families. We have found that clinicians who are certified in the expressive art therapies are typically unfamiliar with some of the interventions and approaches used in play therapy, and vice versa. Therefore, we hope this book will be a bridge between the expressive art therapies and play, as they are therapeutic modalities utilized with children that are complementary in their healing and creative capacities. Play therapists who utilize techniques from the expressive arts disciplines may benefit from exposure to the diverse and innovative approaches within the expressive arts literature that this book presents.

We hope that, after reading this resource book, child and adolescent mental health clinicians, play therapists and clinical supervisors, graduate students in mental health programs, and university educators will become interested in—or in some cases, maybe even become aware of for the first time—a specific expressive art area(s) and seek training or supervised practice to competently employ it with children. This was our singular passion behind writing this project. Although neither Athena nor I claim to be experts in expressive arts, we are licensed mental health clinicians and Registered Play Therapist-Supervisors (RPT-S) who integrate expressive art therapy interventions into our clinical work with children and families. With this transparency and humility, we sought the originators/creators of the distinct areas of the expressive arts, or the leading U.S. authorities in their respective expressive art therapy modalities, to contribute chapters on the subject matter. The contributors comprise a diverse geographic pool across the United States. By utilizing contributors who are leading scholars from the expressive arts and play therapy disciplines, the book presents a unique crossover appeal to clinicians who have one foot in one of the disciplines and want to plant their foot in the other.

This book consists of two introductory chapters. The first chapter highlights the history and spectrum of the expressive art therapies, by one of the leading gurus in the expressive arts therapy field. The second chapter gives an overview of play therapy and its integration of expressive arts interventions through the lens of four major theories. The book then delves into the major disciplines of the expressive arts as distinct chapters. It covers the wide spectrum of art, drama, sandplay, dance/movement, music, photography, and poetry. The book concludes with three chapters integrating the disciplines, specifically in play therapy treatment, for clinical and educational settings.

All of the chapters focus on explicating the respective expressive art therapy modality in a clear, straightforward manner, along with case examples and applications. The majority of the chapters offer practical techniques that can be safely and ethically applied so that clinicians, students, and educators can use this book as a resource to augment their clinical practice. Each chapter also contains information about becoming credentialed in the respective discipline. A resource appendix appears at the end of each chapter to illustrate the systematic nature of simultaneous curricular and supervised experiential training required with all of the respective expressive art therapy disciplines.

One of the core concerns in writing this book was the attention to and mindfulness required by child-based clinicians of ethical and supervision implications in practicing outside one's training and scope of practice. This book seeks to address cross-disciplinary core competency issues while offering clinicians practical ways to apply expressive arts techniques to further enhance their treatment modality with children and families. Readers are urged to seek outside supervision regarding use of applications from disciplines beyond their training. Also, this book is by no means a substitute for what constitutes best practices when learning new areas within the field of mental health counseling: formal education/training, supervised practice, and critical reflectivity/therapist-initiated inner work. The significance of engaging in ongoing reflectivity in our archetypal role as the "wounded healer" expands our collective awareness and calls us to be responsible, progressive, and endlessly curious. The childlike *puer aeternus* calls us to forgo complacent behaviors and to seek new aspects of our field, new paradigms validated by research, and new paths to take that may lead us to understandings of ourselves and our patients that could deepen our work with them.

In conclusion, we hope that readers will find comfort and creativity in this book and that it will enrich their child mental health treatment protocol. Last, we honor the paths already illuminated by those who have paved the way before us in these rich traditions of helping others to self-heal through creative media. May all of our work become more interdisciplinary and inclusive. And may we all contribute to cross-fertilization—where the expressive arts, replete with all of its equally important and numerous disciplines, are accessible and beneficial to those very children who need them the most. Let us now "play on," and begin the journey of this book.

Eric J. Green
Athena A. Drewes

Acknowledgments

First and foremost, we'd like to thank our editor, Rachel Livsey, from John Wiley, for believing in this project from the very beginning. Rachel, you were so supportive of this project from its inception that you illuminated the path for it to come to fruition. Thank you for all of your tireless efforts, for your encouragement, for your editorial acumen, and for believing.

We'd also like to thank Eliana Gil, who was consulted very early on and helped the book take shape and focus. Thank you, Eliana, for your selfless contributions behind the scenes that went into helping us envision this book.

Barry M. Cohen, ATR-BC (Expressive Therapies Summit; www .expressivetherapiessummit.com), you were hugely instrumental in the formation of the content of this book, its focus, and securing the appropriate scholars in their respective disciplines. Thank you for your support and guidance!

We also want to thank all of the contributors of the chapters. It was a humbling experience working with each of you, as you are gurus and legends in your own right. Thank you for your incredible contributions to this volume. Let us all rejoice that we are working together to continue the literature in support of integrative treatment for children and families from the expressive art therapy framework!

And finally, we want to thank all of you, the readers, who support and understand the utility of the expressive arts and the curative power of play therapy to help children and families heal. May this book be a part, however small, in assisting you along the journey in deepening your meaningful and valuable work with children.

Eric J. Green
Athena A. Drewes

About the Editors

Eric J. Green, PhD, LPC-S, RPT-S, LMFT, Certified School Counselor (K–12), is Associate Professor of Counseling at the University of North Texas at Dallas and is also a part-time faculty member and coordinates the annual play therapy institute at the Johns Hopkins University in Baltimore, MD. He has more than 50 professional publications related to children's mental health, including book chapters, magazine submissions, and peer-reviewed journal articles on play therapy and child-related trauma. He is the author of the upcoming book, *Handbook of Jungian Play Therapy* (Johns Hopkins University Press), as well as the film, "Jungian Play Therapy and Sandplay" (Alexander Street Press). Dr. Green is a frequently invited speaker at Association for Play Therapy (APT) state branch conferences across the U.S. and internationally. In 2013, some of his keynote speaking events included the Hawaii Association for Play Therapy Annual Conference in Honolulu, Hawaii; the Australia Pacific Play Therapy Association's Annual 2013 Conference in Gold Coast, Queensland, Australia; and the Canada Association for Child and Parent Therapy 2013 Annual Conference in Niagara Falls, Ontario, Canada. Counselors for Social Justice, a division of the American Counseling Association, presented Eric the O'Hana Award in 2007 and the Mary Smith Arnold Anti-Oppression Award in 2013 for his sustained contributions in mental health advocacy for child trauma survivors. He maintains a part-time, private practice in child and family psychotherapy in Dallas, TX. For more information, visit www.drericgreen.com

Athena A. Drewes, PsyD, RPT-S is a licensed child psychologist, certified school psychologist, and Registered Play Therapist and Supervisor. She is Director of Clinical Training and APA-Accredited Doctoral

Internship at Astor Services for Children & Families, a large multi-service nonprofit mental health agency in New York. She has over 30 years of clinical experience in working with sexually abused and traumatized children and adolescents in school, outpatient, and inpatient settings. Dr. Drewes has worked over 17 years with therapeutic foster care children in treatment. Her treatment specialization is children with complex trauma, sexual abuse, and/or attachment issues.

She is a former Board of Director of the Association for Play Therapy (2001–2006) and Founder/Past President of the New York Association for Play Therapy (1994–2000) and its newly elected President. She has written extensively about play therapy, with seven edited books, and has been a sought-after invited guest lecturer throughout the U.S., England, Wales, Taiwan, Australia, Ireland, Argentina, Italy, Denmark, Mexico, and Canada on play therapy

About the Contributors

Sinem Akay, MS, MEd, LPC-Intern, is a doctoral candidate at the University of North Texas counseling program with a specialization in play therapy. Sinem received a Fulbright scholarship after pursuing her master's degree in clinical psychology in Turkey, and moved to the United States for master's and PhD degrees in counseling. She has advocated for children throughout her education and provided counseling services in the community and schools. Sinem's primary area of scholarship includes play therapy for children with perfectionism and chronic illnesses. Sinem also served as Student Director for Texas Association for Play Therapy (TAPT) and Secretary for the North Texas Chapter of TAPT.

Jennifer N. Baggerly, PhD, LPC-S, RPT-S, is a professor and the Chair of the Division of Counseling and Human Services at the University of North Texas at Dallas. She is Chair-elect of the Board of Directors of the Association for Play Therapy (APT). Jennifer is a Licensed Professional Counselor Supervisor and a Registered Play Therapist Supervisor. She has provided play therapy for 18 years in schools and community agencies and teaches play therapy on a regular basis. Dr. Baggerly's multiple research projects and over 50 publications have led to her being recognized as a prominent play therapy expert.

Sue Bratton, PhD, LPC-S, RPT-S is Professor and Director, Center for Play Therapy, University of North Texas. Dr. Bratton is a nationally and internationally known speaker and author with over 65 publications in the area of play therapy and filial therapy, the majority of which are outcome research. Her most recent books are *Child Parent Relationship*

Therapy (CPRT), CPRT Treatment Manual, Child-Centered Play Therapy Research: The Evidence Base, and *Integrative Play Therapy*. Dr. Bratton is a Past President of the Association for Play Therapy, recipient of the 2007 APT Outstanding Research Award, 2011 CSI Outstanding Supervisor Award, 2013 ACA Best Practice Award, and 2013 AHC Humanistic Educator/Supervisor Award.

Julia Byers, EdD, LMHC, ATR-BC, is currently a professor and Graduate Art Therapy Program Coordinator, co-chair of the Advanced Professional Certificate in Play Therapy, and PhD Senior Advisor in the Interdisciplinary Studies degree at Lesley University, Cambridge, Massachusetts. With over 35 years of clinical practice, university teaching, and administration, Julia has provided Art/Play Expressive Crisis Intervention Counseling in over 18 countries.

Rebecca C. Chalmers, PsyD, MFA, is a published poet, a clinical psychologist practicing in New York City and Brooklyn, and a full-time faculty member at Brooklyn College, City University of New York (CUNY), in the Department of Psychology, where she teaches psychotherapy, psychopathology, and group processes. She specializes in facilitating, and training others to facilitate, Creative Writing Therapy groups and workshops that focus on strengthening mindfulness, preventing clinician burn out, and enhancing creativity.

Jodi Crane, PhD, LPCC, NCC, RPT-S, is Associate Professor in the School of Professional Counseling at Lindsey Wilson College (Kentucky), where she has been teaching for the past 13 years. She received her play therapy training at the University of North Texas. She is the author of chapters in Gary Landreth's *Innovations in Play Therapy* and R. Van Fleet and L. Guerney's *Case Studies in Filial Therapy* (with Sue Bratton). She is the first recipient of APT's Research Grant to complete and publish her research in the *International Journal of Play Therapy*. She serves on the Board of Directors of APT and is a Past President of the Kentucky Association for Play Therapy. In 2010, she received the Terry Fontenot Play Therapy Award for her service to play therapy in Kentucky.

Harriet S. Friedman is on the teaching faculty of the Jung Institute of Los Angeles. She also served at the Jung Institute as director of the Hilde Kirsch Children's Center, serving both parents and children. Harriet is a founding member of the Sandplay Therapists of America (STA), serving STA as Board Chair and having served on the board for the International Society of Sandplay Therapists. Along with Rie Rogers Mitchell she co-authored the book, *Sandplay: Past, Present and Future* (Routledge, 1994) and *Supervision of Sandplay Therapy* (Routledge, 2007). For the last 25 years she has lectured both nationally and internationally on integrating sandplay and Jungian psychology. She has a private practice in West Los Angeles.

Sandra Graves-Alcorn, PhD, LPAT, is founder of the Master's program in Art Therapy and Institute in Expressive Therapies at University of Louisville and a Professor Emeritus at the University of Louisville. Also, she is the Past President of the American Art Therapy Association. Currently, she's in private practice in LaGrange, Kentucky.

Susan Hadley, PhD, MT-BC, is professor of music therapy at Slippery Rock University, Pennsylvania. Her books include *Experiencing Race as a Music Therapist: Personal Narratives* (2013), *Feminist Perspectives in Music Therapy* (2006), and *Psychodynamic Music Therapy: Case Studies* (2003). She co-edited *Therapeutic Uses of Rap and Hip Hop* (2012) and *Narrative Identities: Psychologists Engaged in Self-Construction* (2005) with George Yancy. She has published numerous articles, encyclopedic entries, chapters, and reviews in scholarly journals and academic books. Dr. Hadley serves on the editorial boards of several journals and is co-editor-in-chief of the online journal, *Voices: A World Forum for Music Therapy.*

Dr. Eleanor Irwin, one of the co-founders of the NADT, is also a Child and Adult Psychoanalyst, a Clinical Psychologist, and a TEP Psychodramatist. In addition to being a Clinical Assistant Professor of Psychiatry at the University of Pittsburgh, she is also a Past President of The Pittsburgh Psychoanalytic Center and serves as the Chair of the Child Analysis Committee. She has made films about Expressive Arts

Therapies and has published articles and book chapters about assessment and treatment issues. With Dr. Judith Rubin, she is a co-founder of Expressive Media, Inc., a non-profit organization dedicated to teaching and training in the Expressive Arts Therapies.

Diane Kaufman, MD, is the guiding leader of Creative Arts Healthcare— *The* University Hospital. She is a Child Psychiatrist and Master Clinician at the Rutgers Health Sciences Campus at Newark. She was honored with the Healthcare Foundation of New Jersey's Leonard Tow Humanism in Medicine Award (2000) and Lester Z. Lieberman Humanism in Healthcare Award (2011). Dr. Kaufman is a published poet, an expressive arts educational facilitator with expertise in poetry as therapy, and author of *Cracking Up and Back Again: Transformation Through Poetry*, and the children's story on trauma and resilience, *Bird That Wants to Fly*. She presents internationally on arts and healing.

Mariah Meyer LeFeber, MA, LPC, BC-DMT, DTRL, is a dance/movement therapist and licensed professional counselor at the Hancock Center for Dance/Movement Therapy in Madison, Wisconsin. She currently works with a variety of ages and diagnoses, although her work on dance/movement therapy and children with autism has been published several times. In addition to her work as a therapist, Mariah teaches modern dance and organizes a community outreach and education program in the dance department at the University of Wisconsin, Madison. She enjoys performing as a modern dancer and dancing for joy's sake with her husband and two little girls.

Reina Lombardi, MA, ATR-BC, is an art therapist at Delta Family Counseling in Cape Coral, Florida, and at the Knox Academy in Bonita Springs, Florida. She has 10 years of experience working with children in a variety of residential, clinical, and educational settings. She blends client centered and cognitive-behavioral approaches with the expressive therapies in her work with children. Currently, Mrs. Lombardi serves on the board of the Florida Art Therapy Association and as the Social Media Coordinator for the Expressive Therapies Summit.

Dr. Rie Rogers Mitchell is a professor of educational psychology and counseling at California State University at Northridge, where she serves as clinical director and supervisor at the university's clinic. Dr. Mitchell has been the recipient of several awards at her university, including the University Distinguished Teaching Award and the Dorsey Award for mentoring students in the Educational Opportunity Program. The American Board of Professional Psychology has also awarded her Diplomate status in Counseling Psychology. Dr. Mitchell is a certified sand play therapist and has taught sand play around the world. She has recently been elected President of the International Society of Sandplay Therapists.

Wendy Rosenberg, M.Ed., has been a special educator working with children of all ages for over 20 years. She has brought her love of poetry and poetry therapy techniques into the classroom as well as into homeless shelters, after-school programs, and bereavement workshops. Ms. Rosenberg was the recipient of a Dodge Foundation teacher scholarship to the Fine Arts Work Center. She is a published poet, an Expressive Arts Educational Facilitator, a Certified Applied Poetry Facilitator, a member of the National Association for Poetry Therapy, and a certified Kaizen-Muse Creativity Coach.

Nicole Steele, MT-BC, is a music therapist at the Children's Hospital of Pittsburgh of UPMC, Pittsburgh, Pennsylvania. She received her undergraduate degree in music therapy from Slippery Rock University, Pennsylvania. She has presented at national and regional music therapy conferences as well as medical conferences including the International Transplant Nursing Society Conference.

Dr. Dalena Dillman Taylor is an assistant professor at the University of Central Florida and a Licensed Professional Counselor-Intern. She has extensive clinical experience with play therapy with children, siblings, and families in agencies and schools. She is passionate about the advancement of the counseling field and works to advocate for both the profession and her individual clients. She served as the North Texas

Chapter President of the Texas Association for Play Therapy (2012–2013) and is the recipient of the 2012 SACES Emerging Leader Award.

Professor Robert Wolf is a creative art therapist and psychoanalyst with over 35 years of experience in private practice and clinical supervision. He has been on the graduate faculty of The College of New Rochelle, Pratt Institute, and The Training Institute for the National Psychological Association for Psychoanalysis. He is a former Director of the Institute for Expressive Analysis and a past President of the New York Art Therapy Association. He has published numerous professional articles on art therapy, countertransference, expressive therapy, and phototherapy and his work as a fine art sculptor and photographer have been exhibited internationally.

CHAPTER

1

The Expressive Arts Therapy Continuum: History and Theory

Sandra L. Graves-Alcorn and Eric J. Green

INTRODUCTION

What are the expressive therapies, and what important clinical information do they contextualize for the creative practitioner? In my opinion, we become therapists and utilize expressive art therapies to help others make changes in their lives and guide them toward happier and more fulfilling existences. There are many avenues within the therapeutic milieu to achieve this end. Although the theoretical foundations are often similar, the methods of caregiving to our clients change with our training and chosen area of expertise. Becoming an expressive art therapist and play therapist with children requires accumulating an arsenal of diverse, creative strategies to help clients communicate their experiences and feelings in nonverbal, less threatening ways. It also requires

---

I was very pleased to be asked to write this chapter and thank the editors for the opportunity. I am approaching it partially as personal history and the early development of art therapy as a profession. I was privileged to be among the pioneers and founders of a very important journey in the progress of medical science and healing by use of the expressive arts.

competency based on specified training, credentialing, supervised practice, and ongoing professional development.

Traditional talk therapy alone is generally unsuccessful when working with children and adolescents, especially within the developmental context of young childhood (Green, 2010). Play is a child's work. Toys are their words and play is their language (Landreth, 2012). As an adult, play becomes a necessary balancing act to mitigate typical psychosocial stressors, often bringing out the "natural child" in each of us. Within the venue of play, we find multimedia and multidisciplinary fields. That is not to say that all of the expressive, creative therapies are a form of play therapy, especially given the credentialing and specificity of studies in each professional arena, but for the sake of simplicity and also as a rationale for why we are integrating these fields in this book, I am going to approach integration by highlighting the similarities. I will be explaining the Expressive Therapies Continuum in this chapter as an attempt to lay a foundation of synthesis so all of the therapies can be understood as simply as possible and to formulate a way for the clinician to plan treatment based on integrated theories.

The following definitions of four of the separate disciplines—art therapy, music therapy, drama therapy, and dance therapy—will lead us to what they all have in common and what differences need to be learned in order to be an effective therapist. For the professional standards and criteria, refer to the Specialized Training and Resources section at the end of most chapters for a list of websites and credentialing processes. The information contained in the following four paragraphs was adapted from Expressive Therapy (2013):

> Art Therapy, sometimes called creative arts therapy or expressive arts therapy, encourages people to express and understand emotions through artistic expression and through the creative process. Art therapy provides the client-artist with critical insight into emotions, thoughts, and feelings. Key benefits of the art therapy process include: (a) self-discovery, (b) personal fulfillment, (c) empowerment, (d) relaxation and stress relief, and (e) symptom relief and physical rehabilitation.

> Music Therapy is one of the expressive therapies consisting of an interpersonal process in which a trained music therapist uses

music to help clients improve their psychological functioning, cognitive functioning, motor skills, emotional and affective development, behavior and social skills, and quality of life. Music therapists employ (a) free improvisation, (b) singing, (c) songwriting, (d) listening to and discussing music, and (e) moving to music to achieve treatment goals and objectives. Music therapy is used in some medical hospitals, cancer centers, schools, alcohol and drug recovery programs, psychiatric hospitals, and correctional facilities.

Dance-Movement Therapy (DMT), or Dance Therapy, is the psychotherapeutic use of movement and dance that influences emotional, cognitive, social, and behavioral forms of functioning. As an expressive therapy, DMT assumes that movement and emotion are directly related. The purpose of DMT is to find a healthy balance and sense of wholeness. DMT is practiced in places such as mental health rehabilitation centers, medical and educational settings, nursing homes, day care facilities, and other health promotion programs.

Drama Therapy is the use of theatre techniques to facilitate personal growth and promote mental health. Drama therapy is used in a wide variety of settings, including hospitals, schools, mental health centers, prisons, and businesses. The modern use of dramatic process and theatre as a therapeutic intervention began with Psychodrama. The field has expanded to allow many forms of theatrical interventions as therapy, including role-play, theatre games, group-dynamic games, mime, puppetry, and other improvisational techniques.

MEDIA DIMENSION VARIABLES

In my early pioneering years, I was struck by how expressive arts media had a direct effect on the healing process. So I went about exploring through scientific inquiry and developed what became known as *Media Dimension Variables*, which later transmuted into the *Expressive Therapies Continuum*. I will briefly overview my seminal research in the expressive arts field. Next, I will explain how the media from each expressive arts therapy field can have similar characteristics developmentally and how to incorporate this data clinically.

Early on I defined the use of art and craft materials in therapeutic ser-vice as an exploitation of media dimension variables (MDV) (Graves, 1969). MDV were those qualities or properties inherent in a given medium and process utilized in a therapeutic or educational context to evaluate and/or elicit a desired response from an individual (Kagin, 1969). The premises on which the concept of MDV were developed were that (a) the reinforcement value of making art is inherently a therapeutic process; (b) all individuals can be creative to some degree; (c) dimensions of art media are discernible and can be classified; and (d) media dimensions can be therapeutically applied.

Creativity elucidates a modification of behavior. Creativity, therefore, is a compilation of unconscious and/or conscious information chan-neled into some overt action (Kagin, 1969). A type of cause-and-effect relationship transpires when individuals engage in creative processes that are based on an energy source (motivation) and a data retrieval system leading to problem solving. This original concept was, at that time, based on Guilford's (1965) model for creative performance, which encompassed a need for individuals to experience achievement or self-esteem, a need for expression, and a need for producing order (homeo-stasis in the organism). This creativity was determined by the efficiency with which an individual was able to bring schemata, or information, out of storage for indirect use in coping with situations. Guilford (1965) further divided memory storage into various classes, one of which was visual-figural data, which we see manifest in graphic expression as line, form, and shading.

Art is generally thought to be a socially acceptable mode of creative performance, which may provide enough satisfaction to channel other-wise destructive and/or antisocial actions into constructive and appro-priate channels, as well as alleviate emotional distress. There is an unconscious attempt by an individual when creating art to build sche-mata. This process increases environmental awareness and heightens self-esteem, thus aiding the efficiency with which schemata are used. Ultimately, art making can be viewed as a perpetuating creative cycle (Kagin, 1969).

The theoretical underpinnings of art therapy in the early years of its professional development were that the projections of unconscious material, aided by the spontaneity of graphic expression, would assist the client to gain awareness and insight into inner conflicts that needed resolution. Little attention was given to the media by which these projections were promoted. I, therefore, began looking at specific properties of art media and attempted to hypothesize general emotional or other behavioral responses.

No attention had been given in the literature to different responses when directions were given or not given on the subject or use of the media, or how difficult and complex a project might be and whether it would therefore be suitable for any one individual or group. I also was looking at the physical properties of media, such as fluidity, malleability, indestructibility, expansiveness, unpredictability, and adaptability. Three generalized variables were delineated: (1) structure, (2) task complexity, and (3) media properties.

Media whose properties were soft, aqueous, malleable, and easy to manipulate, such as finger paint, soft clay, polymer acrylics, and so on, were in the fluid range. Resistive materials were defined as hard, brittle, slightly pliable to nonmalleable, and difficult to manipulate, such as hard or highly gorged clay, metal, wood, poster boards, heavier papers, pencils, and so on. A project was considered of high complexity when three or more sequential steps were required for completion, not to include simple repetition of a single process (such as pounding a nail), or of low complexity if the project required only one or two steps.

The difference between the structured and unstructured projects was primarily one of direction. The unstructured goals for completion were left up to the individual, and the instructions were simple (e.g., "Paint anything you wish," "Put the metal on the board in any design you like"). The structured task was presented in a manner designed to leave little, if any, choice in the results of manipulating the materials. Specific directions on how to use the materials resulted in what would be achieved.

The following MDV examples survived not only my thesis study, but also continued on to become part of the curriculum of the Art Therapy Master's degree at the University of Louisville and then an integral and defining element in the Expressive Therapies Continuum (ETC). It is therefore important to understand these combinations and concepts.

When I taught the Methodology lab, I required students to use index cards and a portfolio to dissect each intervention into the MDV, ETC, description of materials used, the procedure and directions for each project, its rationale targeting specific populations or areas of concern to the therapeutic process, and personal reflections as the project affected the student.

Here are some examples from the original projects of my study, which questioned whether different media variables affected verbal communication. Each project was first demonstrated to each participant. The demonstration may or may not be necessary, depending on the person doing the project and the rationale for using it. I am including the instructions and description of materials because it is important that the best media you can afford is used. Many experiences fail for lack of quality media or specificity of instructions. For the sake of space and to remain focused on this chapter's aim, I am including only three of the variables (Potter's Wheel Pot, Mosaic, and Cut and Paste).

Potter's Wheel Pot: HCSF
(High-Complexity Structured Fluid)

Materials included a half-pound of Amaco terra cotta clay, a pan of water, clay sponges, and an electric potter's wheel with a knee treadle. Throwing a pot generally requires a great deal of skill and craftsmanship. However, a reasonable facsimile (clay has roundness and a hole in the middle) is satisfactory. A round ball of white stoneware clay was given to the participant and placed in the center of the wheel's turntable. The therapist formed the original ball to ensure some measure of success. The midpoint was to be found by the participant and corrected until accurate. The therapist then assisted the individual in putting pressure with both hands to the top of the clay mound and pushing it down to enable adherence to the metallic turntable. The wheel was then turned and pushed to top speed, at which time the participant applied pressure to the clay from each side, squeezing in slightly with both palms held rigid and steady in an attempt to establish the center of the clay in the exact center of the wheel. Once the clay was centered as close as possible, both thumbs were placed on center top of the mound and quickly pushed straight down to begin the opening process. The hands are then placed on each side to finish the pot.

Mosaic: HCSR (High-Complexity Structured Resistive)

Material included 30 one-inch-square enameled ceramic tiles (10 red, 10 black, 10 yellow), one pair of tile cutters, an 8-ounce bottle of Elmer's Glue, a 5-inch-by-5-inch piece of pressed board, and a No. 2 drawing pencil. The instructions were to quickly draw lines that would divide the board into at least three areas and thus create a simple design. To color in the design, the tiles were to be glued onto the board in any desired area, and written into the chosen spaces as "R" (red), "B" (black), or "Y" (yellow). The tiles could be broken into smaller pieces by the cutter to enable filling in a smaller area.

Cut and Paste: LCSR (Low-Complexity Structured Resistive)

Materials included one red 22-inch-by-24-inch piece of medium-weight construction paper, on which were drawn in pencil 20 amorphic curvilinear forms; one pair of 5-inch steel teachers' scissors; one 22-inch-by-24-inch piece of white Bristol board (two-ply poster board), on which identical forms to the above were outlined with pencil; and one 8-ounce bottle of Elmer's glue. The participants were required simply to cut out the forms on the red paper and glue them onto the appropriate matched form drawn on the white paper.

Verbalizations were considered important in art therapy at that time, as they would lead to insight and problem solving. There was no significant difference between or among the variables as they related to the type of verbalization I was testing. New research in the area of neuroscience now can explain the relationship between talking and making art, or, more specifically, using the art for memory reinforcement and accuracy, and shows that the nonverbal act of drawing about an event has a much greater retention value than talking about an event (Bruck & Melnyk, 2000). However, in 1969, I was focusing on eliciting verbalizations as a measure of success with the combinations of the variables, complexity, structure, and media properties. It was a start.

I was able to develop a course of study that included all of my theoretical background and experiences, as well as promoted the efficacy of both art as therapy and art psychotherapy. In fact, I saw this well-worn argument by other professionals as a continuum of interventions, which allowed flexibility and included a wide range of populations who could benefit from our services. In the early 1970s, I founded the Institute of Expressive Therapies, with the intent to include music, dance, drama, and poetry into the curriculum. This was the beginning of observing the commonalities among the disciplines, rather than the differences. My colleague, Vija Lusebrink, joined the faculty, and together we researched the interrelationships among the various expressive therapies.

We found a commonality first in developmental theory. The well-known work of Viktor Lowenfeld (1952) in the field of art education had long been one of the foundations on which the MDV was founded. Because the field of art therapy was fixing "deviating" behaviors, then what was the "normal" or expected and acceptable behavior in the arts arena? To recognize deviations, you must know the developmental norms. Although other researchers wrote about the development of children's graphic expression, I was especially taken with Lowenfeld (1952) and Piaget (1962, 1969). When the stages were placed side by side, they explained each other coherently. The development of *schema* in particular was of common importance as a pattern of thinking that built upon itself and manifest in drawing behaviors, play behaviors, and development of symbolic language.

Following Piaget's (1962) developmental sequence with use of various arts media, properties, structure (control), and complexity (cognitive understanding), we begin with sensorimotor play, which translated into the Kinesthetic/Sensory level of the continuum. Babies practice play, repeating motions over and over until the action becomes embedded into a form of its own cognition. The Perceptual/Affective level then begins as motion becomes form and touch or other sensory experiences effects feelings. These feelings do not yet have a verbal language, but they begin to serve the function for which they were biologically created. Anger makes change in the immediate present; sadness slows down the body and mind and processes loss; fear alerts us to danger; and happiness or joy balances all of the other experiences and gives motivation for growth. As form begins to develop further into signs, a meaning becomes attached to the action that created the form. Then the Cognitive/Symbolic level is attained.

The stages of Graphic Development may be aligned with Piaget's (1962) development of schema—or a pattern of thinking on which we all build throughout a lifetime. Lowenfeld (1952) also described *schema* as a visual pattern of rules resulting from early scribble behavior, to making concentric movements, to attaining control enough to create form and name it. The scribble stage occurs generally when the child is able to hold an instrument without eating it and purposely put marks on paper (or whatever background may be selected or available). This can begin anywhere from age 12 months to 18 months and is random in nature. When longitudinal scribbling begins, around age 2, the back-and-forth repetition of practice play assumes a purpose, and experimentation into circular motion occurs. When these motions are mastered, around age 3, the form is purposely constructed. The pencil or crayon is lifted off the page and replaced, allowing for other forms to be produced. With more practice and more schema development, these forms become named, and the cephalopod (body/head configuration) is born. This occurs at approximately age 4, and the ability to draw a human figure begins. In the preschematic stage (ages 4 to approximately 6), much practice and change takes place. The forms do not yet have a set pattern and are randomly placed on the page. When a schema develops (about age 7), then the child has a definite manner in which an object or person is drawn and follows his or her own rules for such drawing. As cognition grows and flourishes, so do the drawings. When an experience is important to the child, a schema deviation takes place to allow for the significance of the experience. Realism is then attempted as the child attempts to draw what he or she sees, not just from internal structure of rules, but also from an external awareness that he or she is trying to translate. Realism begins around age 9, which is also the age when most people arrest further development of drawing spontaneously.

How do media enhance or inhibit this development process? Returning to the media properties ranging from fluid to resistive materials, it is by process of entrainment, resonance, and isomorphism that the media affects the motion and the amount of physical, mental, or emotional energy needed to use it. A LCUF (Low-Complexity Unstructured Fluid) project such as finger painting is basically a Kinesthetic/Sensory experience, where the physical properties of the finger paint are given primary emphasis. If one resonates with the fluidity of the finger paint on the wet paper, the experience should elicit a fluid, fairly unrestricted response, much like you would expect from a 3-year-old. Assuming a normal, healthy, unrestricted response, the 3-year-old will play with the paint joyfully and develop a rhythm to create form. What are the other developmental tasks of the 3-year-old? Would these still be valuable in the adult world? Of course, otherwise we would not be using them as therapeutic treatment toward some specified goal! What does it mean if the individual does not like to touch the finger paint, or get dirty, or feels silly, out of control, and so forth? As educated and intuitive therapists, we should know the answers to these questions. Would you purposely give an experience that you knew would create resistance? Maybe. Under what circumstances and why? My point is that we must anticipate the reaction to each variable along each continuum or we are at best floundering and, at worst, doing harm to our clients. Think now of other arts and play forms: movement and dance, sound and music, sandplay, and drama. They follow the same development on the continuum.

If *isomorphism* takes place and the individual becomes attuned to the media, with a clear understanding of the structure (direction), then some emotional response should be elicited. If we go back to the function of emotions, where anger is used to make change, fear to alert to danger, and so on, we begin to see how and why individuals react to the media dimensions and levels of the ETC the way they do. There is an additional factor, a reinforcement value of experiencing the steps and completion of the project that must also be considered. Does the person respond to fluid materials in a resistive manner? Do resistive materials frustrate and make the person angry? How does the person use the anger to make a change? Are the directions given facilitating the functional use of emotions or causing anxiety or fear? What is alerting the individual to a danger signal? Is the project too complicated? Are the materials outside of the personal boundaries of comfort due to temperament, environment, or past experiences? What was the rationale for giving the project, and was the anticipated outcome achieved? If not, why? These questions form the basics of a therapeutic design using the MDV and ETC.

Actions and Metaphors

Materials elicit and absorb action and reaction, enhancing awareness of the mind–body connection. When materials are fluid, they may be described, as in the case of finger paint, as sliding, slippery, sticky, slick, smoothing, petting, runny, smearing, and so on. The sensation may be described as soft, gooey, pasty, tacky, and even yucky. Each of these reactions may be explored for background information or directed toward problem solving or insight, depending on the level of the ETC with which you are working. Fluid materials generally elicit a loose, flowing response, especially when there is no mediator between material and hand (such as a brush or scraper). When you observe the approach to the materials, even before the action is taken, you assess something about the person. Is the usage without hesitation and spontaneous, or more calculated and cautious? Does this relate to temperament or conditioning or both? Look for the metaphors.

When Gestalt Art Therapy was introduced by Janie Rhyne (1996), she approached the process as the self and asked her clients to give the experience a voice, preceding a description of materials, line, form, color, and space with "I am." Although this may work well with late teens or adults by using verbal language to describe the project, it is still a viable theory as a nonverbal form of communication between the media (foreground) and the background on which the media is manipulated. Is the child soothing, smearing, sliding, or did the media elicit slapping, dotting, poking, or testing? If the intent of using a LCUF project with finger paint was to regress or release, did it work? If not, why? These are questions for the therapist to be able to answer.

Boundaries and Cognition

Fluid materials are contained; otherwise, they would be all over the place. One way to place a medium on the continuum is to determine what kind of container it needs and how much needs to be contained. Using the finger paints again, note that when an amount is placed on the paper, it stays where it is placed—not so with tempera paint or inks. Boundaries are either inherent in the materials or must be made by the participant. Internal controls may also be observed. How much paint is put or poured onto the background material? Selection of fluidity or restiveness may speak to the need for, lack of, or too much boundary. Control is another variable that is directly kin to boundary. Persons with few boundaries may also lack control or, conversely, be demonstrating a need for such. Let's go to the other end of the continuum for an example. A High-Complexity Structured Resistive experience usually is found on the Cognitive/Symbolic level, where intellectualization, control, and even obsessive-compulsive needs may be demonstrated. Let's look at the example of an HCSR experience, the mosaic.

In the more complex experiences, several steps have to be considered both separately and collectively. The materials listed for the mosaic are tiles, which are very resistive and contained. They have no malleability unless quite a bit of force is exerted to break them into pieces, or the project is designed to have all of the tiles the same, and then placing becomes the focus. If the client needs to be able to perform action on the materials in an assertive, yet controlled manner, then a mediator is introduced to facilitate control (the hammer), and the tiles are placed on a surface that will absorb the action. If the appropriate amount of pressure is exerted, the tiles will break where they fissure. If too much force is used, the tiles may be smashed to dust or such tiny particles that using them for the mosaic will be very difficult. What is the metaphor here? How does the individual approach a task or problem?

In the case of a child, teaching the limits is important, and then the choice to adhere or not is made. This is actually true of the adult as well. In complex tasks, teaching allows for a sense of mastery. If the individual has never encountered the materials or process before, then a directive such as, "Do anything you wish," which is totally unstructured, will probably raise the anxiety level. However, the purpose of the structure is to give the guidelines and boundaries for the experience, tending to yield the results that have the highest reinforcement value. Hence, each directive is given with each phase of the project.

In the beginning, it is good to go over all of the instructions so the individual may begin to image a finished product, but using each step in a therapeutic manner is very important. Go back to pounding the tiles. Pounding is, as are all actions on materials, metaphorical. Does your client pound, bang, crash, smash, peck, or only touch the hammer to the tile? What step is next? Depending on whether you have required a design before beginning or allowing for the materials and person to dictate the design is another therapeutic decision. Cognitive development comes into play at this point, as well as the rationale for using this project in the first place. What do you wish to emphasize? Usually the HCSR project is very specified, allowing the client to follow clear directives. Deciding how to create the design with the tiles is an excellent interactive tool.

Your assistance as a therapist should fit the needs of the individual. If discriminate learning is a goal for a child, then sorting the tiles according to size needs to be the next step. If the person has developed beyond the schematic/realistic stage, then creating design (which can lead to homeostasis and another metaphor regarding balance and integration) would probably be a good choice. What is *design*? The term needs to be understood by the client, so ask him or her, "How do you want to plan where to put your tiles?" The response should dictate your reaction. If the individual says, "I want to make a landscape," then the next question is, "What kind of landscape and what do you want in it?" There is safety in rules, permitting clients to feel comforted by structure. If the response is more vague, such as, "I want to make a pretty design," then ask the person if he or she already has one in mind, and ask that it be drawn on a separate piece of paper. Following the principle of isomorphism, I like to help the client create space that yields design. I often take a piece of paper and ask the client to use straight lines and curvy lines to divide the paper into three parts, using the lines from one edge of the paper to another. Not only are you helping to divide and assess the space being used, but you are creating boundaries and teaching esthetic balance.

Symbolic Representation and Interpretations

Going back to the developmental cognitive continuum, the ETC begins with the database of knowledge that is conscious and reaches toward the symbolic meaning of configurations. It is very important to integrate all of the levels when wandering into the symbolic territory. The unconscious manifests itself from basic temperament (instinct) to formal operations into latent memories, conflicts, or universal experiences, which yield transformation of body, mind, and spirit. Whether you are working with a young child who uses play to liquidate or compensate for experiences, or a highly talented, intelligent adult who is open to various interpretations of line, form, object, and color, symbolism is the most obtuse or apparent form of communication!

As a child's play is his work (Green, 2010) and an adult's work needs to have an element of play, the meaning and meaningfulness is the healing. Acceptance of the spiritual—that there is significance in the universe and that each person's life is significant and has meaning and purpose—tends to be an awareness that is the end goal in any therapeutic endeavor. Every form of psychotherapy ultimately resounds in a sense of comfort, peacefulness, hope, and a desire to continue living a better life, resulting in the resilience necessary for adaptation. For a child, this is a developmental process, and we hope we have aligned the development to reach its greatest potential. For the teen who is transitioning hormonally and socially, our interventions and connections will foster hope about the adult world and entering into a career path. In early adulthood, and throughout the lifespan development, each milestone that must be achieved and integrated is part of our therapeutic design. When there is a major change in the path and grief is the result of losses, the tools of the creative arts therapist and the concepts of the ETC help establish the resilience needed.

DISCERNING RATIONALE

The choice of materials or projects should rest with the client. A range of fluid to resistive media needs to be available but not overwhelming. I have a set of markers, crayons, oil pastels, and colored pencils in one section of the art table. Tempera or acrylic paints and various sized brushes, along with the newer contained painting tools (no use of brush required), sit next to plates and bowls for mixing as well as cups for water and paper towels. A variety of papers is also available, in different sizes, colors, textures, and so on. Glue and scissors are placed next to wires and string or yarn. Modeling clays and plasticene are set alongside tools for sculpting. My sandtray is on the floor next to the art table, with containers of action figures, animals, people, soldiers, dinosaurs, and so on easily available for sandplay. In a nearby closet are large bins of craft materials, found objects, toys, dolls, stuffed animals, puppets, drums, balls, and more. In a different section of the room are playhouses and a kitchen set. In the adjacent room is a game table, comfortable sofa, and a desk. My "cozy corner" has an electric fireplace, overstuffed chairs, throws, and a large ottoman, which also serves as a toy/object box. The two rooms are actually arranged according to the ETC, with open space for kinesthetic and sensory activities, as well as contained spaces for perceptual/affective to cognitive symbolic activities. The materials range from fluid to resistive on a large table, but they are not cluttered together. Other furniture fulfills the needs for family space, couples facing each other, or privacy. The environment must be conducive to accessing materials, experiences, and atmosphere at all levels and appropriate for different ages.

Begin where your client begins. During evaluation when selection of materials is made, note the levels of the ETC and the variables of the media. Most people are not well-versed in the use of arts media, so a certain amount of awareness induction and teaching needs to take place. I almost always introduce art experiences in terms of emotional metaphors and function. I demonstrate how good it feels if I am angry to pound on the drum or clay. If sadness is predominant, I can soothe with clay, paint, or rhythm. When I want to feel safe and am afraid, I may build a structure with blocks to protect me, or hug the dolls, or even sift through the sand. Through the expressive therapies, we are helping to create a different language, a different perspective and identity. We build on strengths and growth, resilience, and a positive attitude. Art is science, and science is interwoven into our spirit and psyche. We mirror integration, and we meet ourselves through our creations.

REFERENCES

Bruck, M., & Melnyk, L. (2000). Draw it again Sam: The effect of drawing on children's suggestibility and source monitoring ability. *Journal of Experimental Child Psychology, 77*, 169–196.

Expressive therapy. (2013). In *Wikipedia*. Retrieved from http://en.wikipedia
.org/wiki/Expressive_therapy

Graves, S. (1969). "Media Dimension Variables in Art Therapy." Congress of
the American Society of Psychopathology of Expression. Boston, MA.

Green, E. J. (2010). Children's perceptions of play therapy. In J. Baggerly,
D. Ray, & S. Bratton (Eds.), *Effective play therapy: Evidence-based filial and
child-centered research studies* (pp. 249–263). Hoboken, NJ: John Wiley.

Guilford, J. P. (1965). *Creativity in childhood and adolescence*. Palo Alto, CA:
Science and Behavior Books.

Kagin, S. G. (1969). *The influence of structure in painting on verbal and graphic
self-expression of retarded youth* (Unpublished master's thesis). University of
Tulsa, Tulsa, OK.

Landreth, G. (2012). *Play therapy* (3rd ed.). London, England: Routledge.

Lowenfeld, V. (1952). *Creative and mental growth* (2nd ed.). New York, NY:
Macmillan.

Piaget, J. (1962). *Play, dreams, and imitation in childhood*. New York, NY: Basic
Books.

Piaget, J. (1969). *The Psychology of the Child*. NY: Basic Books.

Rhyne, J. (1996). *The Gestalt art experience: Patterns that connect*. Chicago, IL:
Magnolia.

2

Play Therapy

ATHENA A. DREWES AND SUE C. BRATTON

INTRODUCTION

Play therapy is an empirically supported psychotherapeutic treatment for children founded on the developmental and healing properties of play (Bratton, Ray, Rhine, & Jones, 2005; Schaefer & Drewes, 2011). The Association for Play Therapy (APT; 2013) defines play therapy as:

> The systematic use of a theoretical model to establish an interpersonal process wherein trained play therapists use the therapeutic powers of play to help clients prevent or resolve psychosocial difficulties and achieve optimal growth and development. (p. 2)

As seen in this broad definition, play therapy includes a variety of theoretical models that use play *as* therapy, including child-centered play therapy (Axline, 1969; Landreth, 1991), Jungian play therapy (Allan, 1988; Green, 2011), and psychodynamic play therapy. These modalities are primarily nondirective and child-led. Other theoretical models, such as cognitive-behavioral play therapy (Knell, 2003), Adlerian play therapy (Kottman, 2003), prescriptive play therapy (Schaefer, 2003), and ecosystemic play therapy (O'Connor & Ammen, 1997), use play *in* therapy and advocate a more directive or integrated approach.

RATIONALE FOR PLAY THERAPY

Play is essential to children's optimal brain development (Perry, 2001) and, thus, fundamental to children's healthy functioning in social, emotional, cognitive, and physical domains (Brown, 2009). From a neurobiological perspective, then, play is critical for children whose development has been arrested by distressing life events. Historically, the use of play in child therapy is predicated on two main rationales: (1) play, in and of itself, is curative (Schaefer, 1999); and (2) play is the natural means by which children learn about their world and communicate with others (Landreth, 1991).

In play therapy, children are able to express themselves concretely, using play and symbols much in the same way adults use words (Landreth, 1991). Uniquely human, the pretend play of children represents their efforts to make sense of their experiences through symbolism, fantasy, and make-believe (Russ, 2007). Play allows children to communicate to self and others, make meaning of their experiences, and work through distressing and traumatic events within a safe and nurturing relationship (Gil & Drewes, 2005). Through play therapy, the therapist is allowed the opportunity to enter into the child's experience as it is played out (Landreth, 2012) and to facilitate the child's growth and healing in a way that is consistent with development (Reddy, Files-Hall, & Schaefer, 2005). Although typically viewed as a treatment for young children, play modalities have been successfully applied with clients across the lifespan based on the healing and expressive properties of play (Bratton et al., 2005; Schaefer, 2003).

HISTORY AND DEVELOPMENT

Although child psychotherapists have used play as a means of communication with their young clients since the early 1900s, the formation of the Association for Play Therapy (APT) in 1982 established play therapy as a specialized treatment modality within the field of mental health. The APT's influence, along with the development of university-based play therapy training programs and a surge in publications and research, provided the impetus for the rapid growth and development of the field over the past 30 years. Currently, more than 7,000 mental health professionals identify themselves as play therapists who utilize play in some form in their treatment of children and adolescents (APT, 2013). Play therapy has evolved over its long history to include a cluster of treatment methodologies and theoretical schools of thought. The following sections are an overview of the development of the major theoretical models of play therapy.

Psychoanalytic Play Therapy

The use of play in child psychoanalysis as a means for children to express themselves dates back to the early 1900s (A. Freud, 1928; S. Freud, 1909; Hug-Hellmuth, 1921; Klein, 1932). Anna Freud and Melanie Klein have been traditionally acknowledged as the founders of play therapy. In order to apply analytical approaches to their work with children, they used play to replace verbalized free association and to uncover the past. Within the context of a therapeutic alliance, play and toys allowed children to access unconscious thoughts and feelings, much like dreams were used therapeutically for adults. In psychoanalytic play therapy, healing occurs through bringing unconscious conflicts into conscious awareness and strengthening ego (Carmichael, 2006).

Contemporary psychoanalytic play therapists have since moved from treating play mainly as a vehicle for the expression and interpretation of preconscious and unconscious material. Rather, they see the engagement of the therapist with the child directly through play itself as therapeutic (Levy, 2011). Current thinking has now moved into the spheres of relationship and neurobiology, emphasizing the collaborative and individualized co-construction of meaning through a creative engagement between patient and therapist (Levy, 2011).

Release Play Therapy

Release play therapy is an extension of the work of David Levy (Kaduson, 2011). This approach focuses on the treatment of specific problems through simple release (e.g., throwing, pounding, screaming, or spilling, splashing water), release of feelings in standard situations (e.g., family situations, sibling rivalry), and release of feelings in specific situations (e.g., re-creating or facilitating the creation of a situation to express anxieties). Based on a view of play as the medium for healing and change, release play therapy provides a safe, supportive environment in which children can express feelings of anxiety, anger, fear, or other negative reactions through abreactive and cathartic play (Kaduson, 2011).

Child-Centered Play Therapy (CCPT)

Virginia Axline (1947) applied her training as a student of Carl Rogers to her work with children. Axline based her approach on her belief in children's capacity for self-directed healing and the developmental and curative properties of play. She termed her approach *nondirective play therapy*. A colleague of Axline's, Clark Moustakas (1953), developed a similar nondirective approach predicated on his humanistic and existential leanings and called his model *relationship play therapy*. Louise Guerney (1983) and Garry Landreth (2012) built on the efforts of Axline and Moustakas and further popularized what has come to be known as child-centered play therapy (CCPT) in North America. The terms *nondirective play therapy* or *person-centered play therapy* are more commonly used in the United Kingdom and Europe to explain the same underlying belief systems and basic procedures used in CCPT. In CCPT, the therapist provides therapeutic conditions of genuineness, unconditional positive regard, and empathy that, when experienced by children, allows them to experience self-direction, integration, and growth (Bratton, Ray, & Landreth, 2008).

Jungian Play Therapy

John Allan (1988), a trained Jungian analyst, developed Jungian play therapy based on his experience of applying Jungian theory to young clients. The Jungian approach to play therapy emphasizes the importance of the positive therapeutic alliance to activate the self-healing archetype embedded in children's psyches. Within the safety of the therapeutic milieu, children play out their concerns and experiences through the symbolic language of play. The counselor serves as a witness to children's enactments, analyzes play themes, communicates children's struggles and associated feelings in words, and redirects activities to facilitate healing.

Gestalt Play Therapy

Gestalt play therapy originated from Violet Oaklander's (1988) application of Gestalt therapy to children. Gestalt therapy, developed by Fritz and Laura Perls (Perls, 1969) in the 1940s, is a process-oriented mode of therapy concerned with the healthy, integrated functioning of the total organism. Oaklander (2011) emphasized the importance of play as the way that children learn about the world and try out new ways of being more fully themselves within the safety of the therapeutic relationship. The therapist takes an active role to help children work through resistance, strengthen the self, and develop a sense of mastery and control over life circumstances.

Adlerian Play Therapy

Adlerian play therapy (AdPT), developed by Terry Kottman (2003), is founded on Adler's theory that people are indivisible, social, decision-making beings whose actions and psychological movement have purpose (Dinkmeyer, Dinkmeyer, & Sperry, 1987). The children's play reflects their inner characteristics and manner of behavior or style of life (Adler, 1954). In AdPT, the therapist establishes a mutually collaborative relationship with children and helps them gain insight into the goals of behavior, explore alternative perceptions about their life and experience, utilize their goal-directed and purposeful behavior in socially useful ways, and develop more self-enhancing behaviors.

Cognitive-Behavioral Play Therapy

Introduced by Susan Knell (1998), cognitive-behavioral play therapy is based on behavioral and cognitive theories of emotional development and psychopathology. It incorporates cognitive and behavioral interventions within a play therapy paradigm with verbal and nonverbal communication during play activities. Sessions include forming therapeutic goals, having both children and therapist select materials and activities, using play to teach skills and alternative behaviors, having the therapist verbalize the conflicts and irrational logic of the children, and use of praise by the therapist.

Ecosystemic Play Therapy

Ecosystemic play therapy (EPT), developed by Kevin O'Connor (2011), is an integrative model of play therapy grounded in ecosystemic theory and "incorporating key elements of the analytic (A. Freud, 1928; Klein, 1932), child-centered (Axline, 1947; Landreth, 2012), and cognitive-behavioral models (Knell, 1993) of play therapy, as well as elements of Theraplay (Jernberg & Booth, 1999) and reality therapy (Glasser, 1975)" (O'Connor, 2011, p. 33). O'Connor encouraged play therapists "to take a broadly systemic perspective in developing their case conceptualizations and treatment plans" (p. 253). EPT uses theory to match a wide array of techniques and creative interventions to tailor treatment plans to specific clients and their problems. The clinician is required to consider the children, their developmental level, their problems, and the therapy process within the framework of the children's ecosystem. EPT focuses primarily on helping child clients function optimally in the contexts in which they live.

Prescriptive Play Therapy

Prescriptive play therapy, originated by Charles Schaefer (2003), is based on the premise of differential therapeutics (Frances, Clarkin, & Perry, 1984) and holds that some play interventions are more effective than others, for certain types of disorders (Schaefer, 2003). Thus, a child who does poorly in one type of play therapy may do well with another. There is no one size fits all approach (Schaefer, 2003, p. 307), whereby one theoretical school of thought is sufficient to make change across the various and complex identifiable disorders. The prescriptive approach seeks to find the most effective play intervention for a specific disorder, matching the approach to the unique needs of the individual client. The prescriptive approach utilizes eclecticism, selecting from various theories and techniques to create a therapeutic strategy that is best for a particular child.

Filial Therapy

Filial therapy is a play therapy approach in which mental health professionals train and directly supervise parents and other significant caregivers in the principles and procedures of CCPT to use with their own children. Bernard and Louise Guerney developed this innovative approach in the early 1960s, based on their belief that by training and supervising parents to use CCPT skills in special playtimes with their children, the potential for long-term change was enhanced (B. Guerney, 1964). The use of filial therapy approaches by clinicians has grown rapidly over the past two decades, largely because of Landreth's development of a condensed 10-session model, more recently termed Child-Parent Relationship Therapy (CPRT; Landreth & Bratton, 2006). CPRT's strong research base and its use of a manualized treatment protocol (Bratton, Landreth, Kellum, & Blackard, 2006) have contributed to the growing acceptance and use of filial therapy as an effective treatment modality for children presenting with a wide range of problems.

EMPIRICAL SUPPORT

Dating back to the 1940s, play therapy has a lengthy history of research to support its use. A review of outcome studies on play therapy reveals ample evidence that play therapy is an effective treatment for a variety of socioemotional disorders (Bratton & Ray, 2000; Bratton et al., 2005; Ray & Bratton, 2010), with a marked increase in well-designed controlled play therapy studies over the past two decades (Ray & Bratton, 2010). As in most psychotherapy research, play therapy outcome studies are hindered by small sample size. Meta-analysis overcomes this limitation by statistically combining treatment effect sizes from individual studies to examine overall effectiveness.

Results from meta-analytic reviews of controlled play therapy outcome research (Bratton et al., 2005; LeBlanc & Ritchie, 2001; Lin & Bratton, in review) indicate that play therapy demonstrates moderate to large treatment effects across presenting issues and with diverse ethnic and cultural groups. Bratton et al. (2005) conducted the largest meta-analysis to date ($n = 93$) and reported that play therapy interventions produced large positive effects on treatment outcomes for children (mean age = 7 years) across treatment modalities (group and individual), age groups (3–16 years), gender, referred versus nonreferred populations, presenting issue (externalizing and internalizing), and treatment orientation (humanistic/nondirective, behavioral/directive). Individual controlled outcome studies demonstrate play therapy's effectiveness in addressing a wide variety of social, emotional, behavioral, and learning problems, including posttraumatic stress disorder, conduct disorder, disruptive behaviors, aggression, anxiety/fearfulness, depression, ADHD, impulsivity, low self-esteem, reading difficulties, academic achievement, and social withdrawal. Research also supports play therapy's cross-cultural effectiveness and its beneficial outcomes with a broad range of populations, including children who have experienced chronic illness, grief and loss, physical/sexual abuse, domestic violence, adoption and attachment disruptions, natural disasters, and life stressors such as divorce and relocation (Bratton et al., 2005; Bratton & Ray, 2000; Drewes, 2006; Ray & Bratton, 2010; Reddy et al., 2005).

PROCEDURES AND APPLICATION

The sheer number of theoretical models of play therapy prevents us from describing the process, procedures, and application of each within the scope of this chapter. We selected four theoretical models—child-centered play therapy (CCPT), Gestalt play therapy (GPT), Adlerian play therapy (AdPT), and cognitive-behavioral play therapy (CBPT)—to review based on their prevalence in the literature and for their diversity in techniques and approach. The selected models range on a continuum from least directive (CCPT) to most directive (CBPT), with GPT and AdPT falling closer to the middle of the continuum. To highlight how expressive arts media can be integrated within the uniqueness of the four approaches, we demonstrate the application of the theoretical model though the use of sand/sandtray.

Child-Centered Play Therapy (CCPT)

CCPT is a manualized treatment modality (Ray, 2011), with an existing body of research spanning over seven decades to support its effectiveness as a developmentally responsive intervention for children exhibiting a range of mental health concerns (Baggerly, Ray, & Bratton, 2010). Based on Carl Rogers' (1951) person-centered theory, CCPT is one of the most frequently used approaches among play therapists who adhere to a specific theoretical approach (Lambert et al., 2007). Axline (1947) first applied person-centered principles to counseling with children and named her approach *nondirective play therapy*. Over the years, CCPT has become the preferred term in North America (Bratton et al., 2008).

Axline (1947) posited eight guiding principles of this approach. These basic tenets emphasize enhancing the therapeutic relationship. Axline noted that the therapist should (1) develop a warm, friendly relationship with the child; (2) accept the child exactly as he is; (3) facilitate an atmosphere of permissiveness so that the child is free to express himself; (4) recognize and reflect the child's feelings in order to help him gain insight into his behavior; (5) honor the child's inherent capacity to solve his own problems; (6) allow the child to direct the therapy; (7) understand that therapy is a gradual process and should not be hurried; and (8) establish only those limits necessary to ground the child in the world of reality and make the child aware of his responsibility within the therapeutic relationship.

Axline (1947) posited that given this therapeutic environment, characterized by unconditional positive regard, empathic understanding, and genuiness on the part of the therapist, children could flourish and develop a well-balanced, actualized personality. Landreth (1991) extended Axline's views into a philosophical stance and life orientation that extends beyond the playroom, describing CCPT, not as a set of techniques, but rather, as "an attitude, a philosophy, and a way of being" (Landreth, 1991, p. 55). CCPT is distinguished from other theoretical models of play therapy by the steadfast belief in children's innate tendency toward growth and maturity and a corresponding belief in children's ability for self-directed healing (Axline, 1947; Landreth, 2012).

On the basis of this philosophy, children in CCPT are provided the freedom to direct their play and fully express their inner world within the limits of a safe and predictable therapeutic relationship (Axline, 1947; Guerney, 1983; Landreth, 2012). CCPT is based on the premise that within this unconditionally accepting relationship, children are free to examine experiences that are perceived as inconsistent with the concept of self and then work toward revising and integrating those experiences (Landreth, 2012). As children feel positively regarded, they are able to behaviorally express and explore incongruent feelings and thoughts through play and symbolic expression. In this self-exploration process, children are able to integrate a new awareness of self and develop their full capacity (Ray, 2011).

In CCPT, toys are considered children's words and play their language. The CCPT playroom contains a wide variety of toys and materials to promote children's self-directed activity as well as facilitate a wide range of emotional expression. Landreth (2012) proposed a comprehensive list of play materials for a fully equipped playroom grouped into three broad categories: real-life toys, acting-out or aggressive toys, and toys for creative expression and emotional release.

Application of CCPT

Because of the unstructured and therapeutic properties of sand and water, Landreth (2012) recommended these items as staple materials in the CCPT playroom. When space allows, a typical playroom (for children approximately 3 to 9 years of age) should contain a sandbox large enough for children to climb inside and provide space for sitting on the edge. Sandbox dimensions are approximately 3 feet by 3 feet and 12 to 14 inches in depth. The sandbox is filled approximately half full of sand to allow ample sand for scooping, sifting, piling, and burying large items. Landreth (2012, p. 164) provided a photograph of a standard sandbox and sand tools used in CCPT. For older children in CCPT, a standard sandtray is recommended. The use of a sandtray with preadolescent children (9 to 13 years of age) is described elsewhere in this book (Chapter 11).

In contrast to the other theoretical models featured in this chapter, the CCPT therapist does not direct or suggest the use of sandplay for a specific purpose. Consistent with CCPT principles and procedures, children self-select sandplay according to their needs and preferences. Because of its unstructured nature and soothing quality, children of all ages tend to use sandplay in one way or another. The brief case example is excerpted from Bratton, Carnes-Holt, and Ceballos (2011) and illustrates how a 6 1/2-year-old boy in CCPT used sandplay to make sense of and integrate his early multiple abandonment experiences. The sandplay sequence occurred after the child had developed a felt-sense of safety, unconditional positive regard, and trust in the therapeutic relationship.

In this case, few specifics were known about the child's experiences prior to 4 years of age.

Sandplay was a favorite activity for Andy. He used the sandbox as a soft and soothing place to lie and suck on a bottle, a place to "be messy," a place to curl up and hide, and most of all, a place for hiding, and sometimes finding, important figures. In sessions 36 through 46, Andy's sandplay became more focused on themes of loss, attachment, and trust. The soothing quality of the sand seemed important in his play. He played out variations of mothers and babies (animal pairs) trying to find each other, with the babies typically buried in the sand and the mothers "searching" for, and sometimes finding, their babies. He consistently chose a baby dolphin to represent himself. Toward the end of this time period, he began to identify a large dolphin as "the mother." In session 42, he handed the mother dolphin to the therapist and said, "find the baby" (the baby dolphin that he had buried deep in the sand). Andy instructed the therapist that the baby was going to be "hard to find" and to "keep looking everywhere." The therapist was careful to allow Andy to lead the play to determine if he wanted the baby found. Over time, it became clear that Andy did not plan for the mother dolphin to find the baby. He made comments like, "no, not there— keep looking," until the session ended. Throughout the play, he took great delight in the therapist (mother dolphin) methodically searching for the baby and never giving up. Andy seemed to be integrating his early experiences (implicit memories) into a positive, explicit memory of being wanted and special, even if mother and baby were never reunited. Integration was indicated by the cessation of the activity in future sessions and a shift in his affect and play. This brief example demonstrates the child's internal wisdom to know what he needed to make sense of his early experience and to begin to integrate those experiences into a congruent sense of self.

Gestalt Play Therapy (GPT)

GPT, developed by Violet Oaklander (1988), is a humanistic, process-oriented approach that is concerned with the integration of the whole child: senses, body, emotions, and intellect (Carroll & Oaklander, 1997). As described in her book, *Windows to Our Children* (Oaklander, 1988), GPT grew out of applying her training as a Gestalt therapist to her work with children. She found that the concepts and principles of Perls' (1969) original theory of conceptualizing adult clients were equally applicable to understanding her young clients. As with Gestalt therapy with adults, the overall goal of GPT is for children to develop an enhanced awareness of self.

Oaklander (2011) emphasized the importance of play as the way that children learn about the world and try out new ways of being more fully themselves within the safety of the therapeutic relationship. The therapist takes an active role to help children work through resistance, strengthen the self, and develop a sense of mastery and control over life circumstances. Oaklander described the process as a therapeutic dance in which children's needs dictate the therapist's decision whether to follow children's lead or serve as a guide or director. The therapist's clinical judgment is based on sensitivity to children's inner world and the therapist's own inner experience.

Although Gestalt play therapy is associated with the use of a variety of projective and expressive techniques, according to Oaklander (2011), the process of play therapy is more important than techniques. The I/Thou relationship, in which the therapist is as authentic as possible, is the foundation of the therapeutic process. Through children's experience of a warm, nurturing, and genuine relationship, they begin to restore healthy organismic self-regulation, integrate all aspects of self, including those parts that were previously rejected, develop an accurate sense of self, and are able to use resources in the environment to get their needs met. The Gestalt play therapist actively works within children's various systems to foster a greater understanding of, and responsiveness to, their needs.

In GPT, a wide variety of toys and expressive media is used to facilitate children's creativity and exploration of self and experience through fantasy as well as to provide a broad range of sensory experiences. Materials and activities include a variety of toys, household items, crafts, paints, various drawing materials, collage, clay, sandtray, water, puppets, creative dramatics, music, musical instruments, metaphors, and dreams (Oaklander, 2011).

Application of GPT

Sand, water, and miniature figures are standard items in the GPT playroom. Oaklander (1988) provided several case examples of structured and spontaneous use of sandtray activities with children. Oaklander suggests a variety of prompts for creating a sandtray that the therapist uses based on an understanding of the child's developmental and therapeutic needs. The therapist can offer a general prompt such as, "Choose any of the items on the shelves and make a scene or picture in the sand." At other times, the therapist chooses figures in order to focus on a specific issue, such as enacting a real situation in the child's life. Oaklander describes working with the sandtray similarly to a drawing or dream. After the scene is completed, the therapist asks the child to describe the scene, tell a story about it, tell what is happening or is about to happen, and so on. The therapist comments on elements of the scene that seem significant and may ask the child to identify with various objects and give the object a voice, an action, or both: "I'd like you to pretend to be the whale and tell me what it's like at the bottom of the ocean." To encourage children to take on the role, it is helpful for the therapist to stay in the metaphor, "So, whale, what's it like at the bottom of the ocean?" The therapist can also ask the child to give the scene a title. Or, the therapist may comment on the process or overall presentation or theme of the sandtray: "Your animal kingdom looks very crowded; I wonder if you feel like that sometimes." "I noticed that you had a really hard time deciding which animal to place at the top of the mountain." Therapists use their inner experience, feelings, and body sensations as clues to the child's inner experience to guide their comments and questions.

Adlerian Play Therapy (AdPT)

Adlerian play therapy follows Adler's (1954) theory that people are indivisible, social, decision-making beings whose actions and psychological movement have purpose (Dinkmeyer et al., 1987). It is an integration of theoretical concepts of individual psychology with the techniques of play therapy (Kottman, 2009). There are several theoretical tenets:

1. People are social beings and have a need to belong.
2. People are self-determining and are creative.
3. Behavior is goal-directed.
4. Reality is experienced subjectively. (Kottman, 2005)

There are four phases to the treatment process. The first requires the building of a therapeutic relationship based on equality with children, based in trust and an equal sharing of power. The goal is to build a partnership with children as they move forward together through the therapeutic process. In this initial stage, the therapist intentionally shares power with the children and follows their lead. Much like child-centered play therapy, the therapist spends time in this initial phase answering questions about therapy, returning responsibility to the children, and setting any necessary limits. The children's metaphoric play is responded to by the therapist through tracking or restating the children's play content to show they are being heard and understood (Ashby & Noble, 2011).

The second phase explores children's lifestyle and preconceived views and distortions about their world and reality. The therapist uses a variety of directive and nondirective techniques to assist in understanding children's lifestyle, through observation of strengths and resources (Ashby & Noble, 2011).

Children's play reflects inner characteristics and manner of behavior or style of life (Adler, 1954). Children are helped to explore alternative perceptions about their life and experience and to utilize their goal-directed and purposeful behavior to move toward their desired goal. The playroom includes toys to assist children to create rapport with the therapist, convey a variety of emotions, role-play situations and relationships that exist in their life, provide a safe environment to test out behavioral and emotional limits, empower their sense of self, advance self-understanding, and improve their self-control and responsibility for their behavior and feelings (Kottman, 2005).

The therapist assesses how effective children are at attaining positive goals and what their subjective experience has been, while considering how the therapist might challenge any faulty convictions or distortions of reality. Children's unhelpful thoughts, feelings, and behaviors are discovered through their patterns of play (Ashby & Noble, 2011).

The third phase is intended to help children gain insight, which is accomplished through a combination of directive and nondirective techniques. The therapist begins to share observations and utilizes metaphors to help children expand these observations beyond the playroom (Ashby & Noble, 2011). Using metaphor, interpretation, and metacommunication, the therapist helps children to gain insight and make connections between their play in the therapy room and the outside world (Ashby & Noble, 2011).

The fourth phase is Reorientation and Reeducation, whereby the therapist's goals are to help children to generate new behaviors outside of the playroom, through developing skills via teaching and practice using modeling, role-playing, and therapeutic metaphors (Ashby & Noble, 2011).

Adlerian play therapy utilizes a variety of expressive arts materials, such as clay, puppets, sandtrays, drawings materials, and storytelling, along with stuffed animals and books for directive and metaphoric play (Daigneault, 1999).

Application of AdPT

The sandtray is frequently utilized in helping to build a relationship, exploring children's lifestyle, helping them gain insight into their lifestyle, and working on reorientation and reeducation (Kottman, 2005). Children may create their own sandtray first, and then the therapist would share inferences about the children's lifestyle through the creation of another sandtray that tries to depict the therapist's understanding of how the children see themselves, others, and the world; the sandtry may also show perception of the children's personality, or it may show an understanding of the parent–child or family relationships.

The sandtray can also be utilized in a more interactive manner, with the therapist and children working together to reframe a problem situation, or depicting a problem and then adding or taking out items to depict a solution. The therapist can also utilize metaphoric storytelling in telling a story designed to help children gain insight, using objects and the sand (Kottman, 2005). But this can also be done interactively, with the therapist and children telling a story together, with the children first putting an object into the tray, creating a sentence or two using the object as an element of the story, and then the therapist choosing an object that will help move the story along, adding a sentence or two using that object. The therapist and children continue to alternate choosing objects and telling a sentence or two that moves the story forward, with the children placing the last object and finishing the story (Kottman, 2005).

Mutual storytelling can also be used, whereby the children tell a story in the tray or create a world in the tray, and the therapist retells the story or redoes the world in a more constructive manner (Kottman, 2005). The sandtray can be used directively to have children make a tray to show their ideal world, self, family, class, and so on. A perspectives tray (or series of trays) can be created depicting a bunch of different ways of viewing a situation or problem, and then the children choose the one they would be willing to try for the following week (Kottman, 2005).

Cognitive-Behavioral Play Therapy (CBPT)

CBPT is based on behavioral and cognitive theories of emotional development and psychopathology. It incorporates cognitive and behavioral interventions within a play therapy paradigm with verbal and nonverbal communication during play activities (Ashby & Noble, 2011). Sessions include forming therapeutic goals, having both children and therapist select materials and activities, using play to teach skills and alternative behaviors, having the therapist verbalize the conflicts and irrational logic to children, and use of praise by the therapist (Knell, 1998). Knell (1998) identified specific characteristics of CBPT: (a) The child is an active participant in the therapy process; (b) CBPT is focused on the child's environment, along with thoughts, feelings, beliefs, and fantasies; (c) CBPT emphasizes figuring out ways to develop adaptive thoughts and behaviors; (d) CBPT is directive, structured, and goal-oriented; and (e) the therapist uses techniques that have been empirically validated (such as modeling; Bandura, 1977) and can be empirically evaluated for effectiveness.

CBPT has four stages: Assessment, Introduction/Orientation, Interventions, and Termination. In the Assessment phase, the children's and parents' perceptions of their children's current level of development and functioning are assessed through observation, parent report, interviewing, play assessment, psychological testing, and therapist-assigned tasks. In particular, the therapist identifies and assesses the children's cognitive distortions and misconceptions (Knell, 2011).

In the Introduction/Orientation phase, the therapist works with children to prepare for therapy via parent consultation, bibliotherapy, and structured tasks from which treatment and therapeutic goals are identified (Knell, 2009). Parents are involved through regular contact for assessment and consultation regarding their children. During the Middle Stage of therapy, interventions are developed to help children develop adaptive responses to problems, circumstances, and stressors utilizing modeling and role-playing with semi-structured play with puppets and toys, art materials, and bibliotherapy. Through the use of puppet play, children can see the therapist model adaptive and helpful behaviors and coping skills through story character or an interactive dialog with a puppet who may share the children's concerns or fears (Ashby & Noble, 2011), and they can then role-play positive coping statements and behaviors that they can utilize during times of distress. Positive reinforcement for shaping of behavior and extinction of negative behaviors (Knell, 1994) is utilized to help children generalize what they have learned in the therapy sessions out into other settings in their environment (school, after-school activities, spiritual settings). The fourth, and final, stage involves preparing children for termination of therapy. The therapist reinforces the changes they have made and may include additional practice in generalizing learning from the play therapy sessions to other sessions as a form of relapse prevention (Meichenbaum, 1985).

CBPT is usually conducted in an office or playroom, which is equipped with play materials, including an array of traditional play therapy toys that can be used directively as well as metaphorically: stuffed animals, art supplies, puppets, dolls, bibliotherapy books, and DVDs and other materials. Treatment may at times take place outside of the playroom or office where children may have specific anxieties or phobias, which are then treated in *vivo*. Expressive arts materials are often utilized in the treatment process depending on the children's needs and to help in gradual exposure and systematic desensitization in dealing with emotionally laden material and in the trauma narrative.

Application of CBPT

Sandtrays can be utilized within CBPT in helping children to create scenarios that can offer therapeutic insight into their world views, cognitive distortions, life events, and problem-solving skills. The sandtray would be used in a directive, therapist-led manner, whereby children would be instructed to create scenes that would help them further explore their life situations. For example, in the case of a traumatic event, children could be directed—at the appropriate time in treatment after rapport has been established and coping strategies and affect regulation techniques are in place—to create on one side of the sandtray how the children felt, or their life was, before they told about their abuse. Then they would be asked to create in the other half of the tray a scene of how they feel now or how their life is now experienced after having told about the abusive situation (Gil, 2006).

The therapist could also utilize the sandtray to have children create a scene of a time when they have experienced conflict with a parent, peer, or regarding parental divorce (or any other type of conflictual or upsetting situation). The therapist would then encourage children to problem solve to see if there might be possible alternative solutions to the scenario. Could a helper be brought in? Could something be said to change the miscommunication? What could the children say to themselves when they feel scared, worried, or angry about the situation (e.g., thought-stopping strategy)? What solution(s) might be possible to help lessen the problem the children or teens may be experiencing? The therapist and clients would discuss which of the strategies might be the best to try out as homework in the following week, and then the clients would report back at the next therapy session about how the strategy went.

CONCLUSION

Play therapy is an empirically supported modality that has evolved over the past century to include a range of theoretical approaches and treatment interventions/techniques that are grounded in the therapeutic and developmental properties of play. As illustrated in the examples, expressive arts materials and activities can be successfully integrated within various theoretical models to align with therapists' theoretical orientation and to best meet the needs of clients.

SPECIALIZED TRAINING AND RESOURCES

Educational Requirements

The Association for Play Therapy (APT), which is a national professional organization in the United States, grants Registered Play Therapist (RPT) and Registered Play Therapist-Supervisor (RPT-S) credentials to licensed mental health professionals with specialized training and experience in play therapy.

Criteria for Registered Play Therapist (RPT)

- License/Certification to engage in either independent or supervised mental health practice, that is current and active
- Must have a Master's or higher mental health degree with completion of APT-designated core graduate coursework
- Must have completed 2 years and 2,000 hours of verified supervised clinical experience (not more than 1,000 hours at the pre-Master's level)
- Must have completed at least 150 hours of play therapy specific instruction, of which only 50 hours may be noncontact, from an APT-approved provider of graduate-level continuing education
- Must have completed at least 500 hours of supervised play therapy experience that included at least 50 hours of play therapy supervision

Criteria for Registered Play Therapist-Supervisor (RPT-S)

- Must meet all criteria listed above for Registered Play Therapist (RPT)
- Must have completed an additional 3 years and 3,000 hours of clinical experience, which must be verified, but need not be supervised by a licensed mental health professional
- Must have practiced at least 3 years after the initial date of state licensure or certification
- Must have completed an additional 500 hours of play therapy experience (from that required above), which must be verified, but need not be supervised by a licensed mental health professional

- State licensure or certification must either (a) allow the therapist to supervise others, or (b) not specifically prohibit the therapist from supervising others
- Must be a state-approved supervisor or have earned at least 24 hours of supervisor training that is not included in the 150 hours of play therapy training

Criteria for Renewal
- All RPT-S must hold current and active state licensure or certification
- Must have completed at least 36 hours of graduate-level continuing education every 3 years after initial approval
- At least 18 play therapy hours, not more than 9 of which may be noncontact hours. Must have at least 2 hours of supervisor training

All forms and complete requirements and fees are available at: www.a4pt.org

REFERENCES

Adler, A. (1954). *Understanding human nature* (W. B. Wolf, Trans.). New York, NY: Fawcett Premier. (Original work published 1927)

Allan, J. (1988). *Inscapes of the child's world.* Dallas, TX: Spring Publications.

Ashby, J. S., & Noble, C. (2011). Integrating cognitive-behavioral play therapy and Adlerian play therapy into the treatment of perfectionism. In A. A. Drewes, S. C. Bratton, & C. E. Schaefer (Eds.), *Integrative play therapy* (pp. 225–240). Hoboken, NJ: Wiley.

Association for Play Therapy. (2013). *About APT.* Retrieved from www.a4pt .org/ps.playtherapy.cfm?ID=1158

Axline, V. (1947). *Play therapy: The inner dynamics of childhood.* Boston, MA: Houghton Mifflin.

Axline, V. (1969). *Play therapy* (rev. ed.). New York, NY: Ballantine Books.

Baggerly, J., Ray, D., & Bratton, S. (Eds.). (2010). *Child-centered play therapy research: The evidence-base for effective practice.* Hoboken, NJ: Wiley.

Bandura, A. (1977). *Social learning theory.* Englewood Cliffs, NJ: Prentice Hall.

Bratton, S., Carnes-Holt, K., & Ceballos, P. (2011). An integrative humanistic play therapy approach to treating adopted children with a history of attachment disruptions. In A. A. Drewes, S. C. Bratton, & C. E. Schaefer (Eds.), *Integrative play therapy* (pp. 341–370). Hoboken, NY: Wiley.

Bratton, S., Landreth, G., Kellum, T., & Blackard, S. (2006). *Child-Parent Relationship Therapy (CPRT) treatment manual: A 10-session filial therapy model for training parents.* New York, NY: Brunner-Routledge. (Includes CD-ROM)

Bratton, S., & Ray, D. (2000). What the research shows about play therapy. *International Journal of Play Therapy, 9*(1), 47–88. doi:10.1037/h0089440

Bratton, S., Ray, D., & Landreth, G. (2008). Play therapy. In M. Hersen & A. Gross (Eds.), *Handbook of clinical psychology, Vol II: Children and adolescents* (pp. 577–625). Hoboken, NJ: Wiley.

Bratton, S. C., Ray, D., Rhine, T., & Jones, L. (2005). The efficacy of play therapy with children: A meta-analytic review of the outcome research. *Professional Psychology: Research and Practice, 36*(4), 376–390.

Brown, S. (2009). *Play: How it shapes the brain, opens the imagination, and invigorates the soul.* New York, NY: Penguin Group.

Carmichael, T. (2005). *Play therapy: An introduction.* Upper Saddle River, NJ: Pearson.

Carmichael, T. (2006). *Play Therapy: An Introduction.* Upper Sadler, NJ: Pearson/Merrill Prentice Hall.

Carroll, F., & Oaklander, V. (1997). Gestalt play therapy. In K. J. O'Connor & L. M. Braverman (Eds.), *Play therapy theory and practice: A comparative presentation* (pp. 184–203). New York, NY: Wiley.

Daigneault, S. D. (1999). Narrative means to Adlerian ends: An illustrated comparison of narrative therapy and Adlerian play therapy. *The Journal of Individual Psychology, 55*(3), 298–315.

Dinkmeyer, D. C., Dinkmeyer, J. D., & Sperry, L. (1987). *Adlerian counseling and psychotherapy* (2nd ed.). Columbus, OH: Merrill.

Drewes, A. A. (2006). Play-based interventions. *Journal of Early Childhood and Infant Psychology, 2*, 139–156.

Frances, A., Clarkin, J., & Perry, S. (1984). *Differential therapeutics in psychiatry.* New York, NY: Brunner/Mazel.

Freud, A. (1928). *Introduction to the technique of child analysis.* New York, NY: Ayer.

Freud, S. (1909). Analyse der Phobie eines fünfjährigen Knaben ("Der kleine Hans") *Jb. psychoanal. psycho-pathol. Forsch*, I, 1-109; GW, VII, pp. 241–377. [Analysis of a phobia in a five-year-old boy. *SE*, 10, 1–149.]

Gil, E. (2006). *Helping abused and traumatized children. Integrating directive and nondirective approaches.* New York, NY: Guilford Press.

Gil, E., & Drewes, A. A. (2005). *Cultural issues in play therapy.* New York, NY: Guilford Press.

Glasser, W. (1975). *Reality therapy.* New York, NY: Harper & Row.

Green, E. J. (2011). Jungian analytical play therapy. In C. E. Schaefer (Ed.), *Foundations of play therapy* (2nd ed., pp. 61–86). Hoboken, NJ: Wiley.

Guerney, B. (1964). Filial therapy: Description and rationale. *Journal of Consulting Psychology, 28,* 304–310.

Guerney, L. (1983). Play therapy with learning disabled children. In C. E. Schaefer & K. O'Connor (Eds.), *Handbook of play therapy* (pp. 419–435). New York, NY: Wiley.

Hug-Hellmuth, H. (1921). On the technique of child analysis. *International Journal of Psychoanalysis, 2,* 287–305.

Jernberg, A., & Booth, P. (1999). *Theraplay: Helping parents and children build better relationships through attachment-based play* (2nd ed.). San Francisco, CA: Jossey-Bass.

Kaduson, H. G. (2011). Release play therapy. In C. E. Schaefer (Ed.), *Foundations of play therapy* (2nd ed., pp. 105–126). Hoboken, NJ: Wiley.

Klein, M. (1932). *The psycho-analysis of children.* London, England: Hogarth Press.

Knell, S. M. (1993). *Cognitive-behavioral play therapy.* Northvale, NJ: Jason Aronson.

Knell, S. M. (1994). Cognitive-behavioral play therapy. In K. O'Connor & C. Schaefer (Eds.), *Handbook of play therapy, Vol. 2: Advances and innovations* (pp. 111–142). New York, NY: Wiley.

Knell, S. M. (1998). Cognitive-behavioral play therapy. *Journal of Clinical Child Psychology, 27,* 28–33.

Knell, S. M. (2003). Cognitive-behavioral play therapy. In C. E. Schaefer (Ed.), *Foundations of play therapy* (pp. 178–191). Hoboken, NJ: Wiley.

Knell, S. M. (2009). Cognitive-behavioral play therapy: Theory and applications. In A. A. Drewes (Ed.), *Blending play therapy with cognitive behavioral therapy: Evidence-based and other effective treatments and techniques* (pp. 117–134). Hoboken, NJ: Wiley.

Knell, S. M. (2011). Cognitive-behavioral play therapy. In C. E. Schaefer (Ed.), *Foundations of play therapy* (2nd ed., pp. 313–327). Hoboken, NJ: Wiley.

Kottman, T. (2003). *Partners in play: An Adlerian approach to play therapy* (2nd ed.). Alexandria, VA: American Counseling Association.

Kottman, T. (2005). *Partners in the sand: Adlerian applications of sand tray play therapy.* Presented at the 22nd Annual Association for Play Therapy International Conference, October 5–8, 2005, Nashville, Tennessee.

Kottman, T. (2009). Adlerian play therapy. In K. J. O'Connor & L. D. Braverman (Eds.), *Play therapy theory and practice: Comparing theories and technique* (pp. 237–282). Hoboken, NJ: Wiley.

Lambert, S., LeBlanc, M., Mullen, J., Ray, D., Baggerly, J., White, J., & Kaplan, D. (2007). Learning more about those who play in session: The National Play Therapy in Counseling Practices Project (phase 1). *Journal of Counseling and Development, 85,* 42–46.

Landreth, G. L. (1991). *Play therapy: The art of the relationship.* Muncie, IN: Accelerated Development.

Landreth, G. L. (2012). *Play therapy: The art of the relationship* (3rd ed.). Muncie, IN: Accelerated Development.

Landreth, G., & Bratton, S. (2006). *Child-Parent Relationship Therapy (CPRT): A 10-session filial therapy model.* New York, NY: Brunner-Routledge.

LeBlanc, M., & Ritchie, M. (2001). A meta-analysis of play therapy outcomes. *Counseling Psychology Quarterly, 14,* 149–163.

Levy, A. J. (2011). Psychoanalytic approaches to play therapy. In C. E. Schaefer (Ed.), *Foundations of play therapy* (2nd ed., pp. 43–60). Hoboken, NJ: Wiley.

Lin, Y., & Bratton, S. (in review). A meta-analysis of child-centered play therapy outcome research. Submitted to *Journal for Counseling and Development.*

Meichenbaum, D. (1985). *Stress inoculation training.* New York, NY: Pergamon Press.

Moustakas, C. (1953). *Children in play therapy.* New York, NY: McGraw-Hill.

Oaklander, V. (1988). *Windows to our children.* New York, NY: Gestalt Journal Press.

Oaklander, V. (2011). Gestalt play therapy. In C. E. Schaefer (Ed.), *Foundations of play therapy* (2nd ed., pp. 171–186). Hoboken, NJ: Wiley.

O'Connor, K. (2011). Ecosystemic play therapy. In C. E. Schaefer (Ed.), *Foundations of play therapy* (2nd ed., pp. 253–272). Hoboken, NJ: Wiley.

O'Connor, K. J., & Ammen, S. (1997). *Play therapy treatment planning and interventions: The ecosystemic model and workbook.* San Diego, CA: Academic Press.

Perls, F. S. (1969). *Ego, hunger and aggression.* New York, NY: Scribner.

Perry, B. (2001). *Maltreated children: Experience, brain development, and the next generation.* New York, NY: W. W. Norton.

Ray, D. (2011). *Advanced play therapy: Essential conditions, knowledge, and skills for child practice.* New York, NY: Routledge.

Ray, D., & Bratton, S. (2010). What the research shows about play therapy: 21st century update. In J. Baggerly, D. Ray, & S. Bratton (Eds.), *Child-centered play therapy research: The evidence base for effective practice*. Hoboken, NJ: Wiley.

Reddy, L. A., Files-Hall, T. M., & Schaefer, C. E. (2005). *Empirically based play interventions for children*. Washington, DC: American Psychological Association.

Rogers, C. (1951). *Client-centered therapy*. Boston, MA: Houghton-Mifflin.

Russ, S. (2007). Pretend play: A resource for children who are coping with stress and managing anxiety. *NYS Psychologist, XIX*(5), 13–17.

Schaefer, C. E. (1999). Curative factors in play therapy. *Journal for the Professional Counselor, 14*(1), 7–16.

Schaefer, C. E. (2003). Prescriptive play therapy. In C. E. Schaefer (Ed.), *Foundations of play therapy* (pp. 306–320). Hoboken, NJ: Wiley.

Schaefer, C. E., & Drewes, A. A. (2011). The therapeutic powers of play and play therapy. In C. E. Schaefer (Ed.), *Foundations of play therapy* (2nd ed., pp. 15–25). Hoboken, NJ: Wiley.

CHAPTER

3

Art Therapy

Reina Lombardi

INTRODUCTION

People have been using the arts as a method of understanding the human spirit and as an agent of healing throughout human history. Evidence of this practice can be found in the Paleolithic cave paintings of Lascaux, France (Leroi-Gourhan, 1982), as well as in the healing practices of shamans in native cultures (Sander & Wong, 1997). Psychiatrists, hailing from various countries, began documenting, examining, and publishing about the artwork created by their patients with mental illness at the beginning of the 19th century (Beveridge, 2001; Hogan, 2001). Perhaps the most notable publication from this time period was by German psychiatrist Hans Prinzhorn, whose book *Artistry of the Mentally Ill*, first published in 1922, documented numerous images of artwork created by individuals with mental illness (Prinzhorn, 1972). Unlike his predecessors, Prinzhorn sought to look at the artwork as products of individuals rather than as a way to substantiate or quantify their illness. During the height of Freudian psychoanalysis, many following the discipline began using art within their practices with patients as a method of accessing and bringing unconscious material to life (American Art Therapy Association, 2012; Junge, 2010; Rubin, 2001a).

Art therapy emerged as a union of the theoretical underpinnings from the fields of psychology and art. Educators and art therapy pioneers,

Margaret Naumburg, Florence Cane, and Edith Kramer, were each influenced by the work of Freud, and they began formalizing the construct of art therapy in the mid-20th century through their work with children (Cane, 1983; Junge, 2010; Kramer, 2000; Rubin, 2001a). Naumburg, who is often thought to be the matriarch of art therapy in America, and Mary Huntoon, who is credited with creating one of the first art therapy studios in the United States, introduced art therapy in their work with adults in psychiatric hospital settings in the early 20th century (Junge, 2010; Rubin, 1999). The profession expanded because of the work of these and other pioneers in the early 20th century, but it took several decades for roots to take hold and mature into the development of collegiate degreed training programs in the late 1950s and the professional organization, the American Art Therapy Association (AATA), in 1969 (Junge, 2010). In an effort to avoid presenting a myopic view of the field, it is important to recognize that as the profession of art therapy was being established in the United States, like-minded innovators were founding the profession abroad (Edwards, 2004; Hogan, 2001; Junge, 2010; Rubin, 1999). Readers interested in learning more may choose to consult Junge's (2010) comprehensive text *The Modern History of Art Therapy in the United States*.

ART THERAPY: THEORY

Theory, specifically its application within clinical practice, is the foundational component to the competent practice of art therapy. It provides a rich, dynamic framework to understand the diverse means in which art therapy can be an effective therapeutic modality (Rubin, 1999, 2001b). The theories briefly covered in this chapter represent only a few of the theories utilized within the field, particularly those that are useful in working with children and adolescents. It is recommended that readers access original source materials to procure a comprehensive understanding of art therapy theory.

Psychoanalytic

The psychoanalytic theories of both Sigmund Freud and Carl Jung have deeply influenced the pioneers of the art therapy field. Margaret

Naumburg (1987) integrated aspects of both Freudian and Jungian theory in her practice of *Dynamically Oriented Art Therapy*, which she explains in her manuscript of the same name. Naumburg's approach focused on unearthing unconscious material through the use of free association about nondirected or spontaneously produced artwork (1987). The goal of free association is to aid the client in developing the intrapersonal insight and understanding that is necessary for change to occur (Malchiodi, 2003; Rubin, 2001a).

Edith Kramer, who was also influenced by psychoanalytic theory, practiced an approach known as *art as therapy* (Kramer, 2000). Kramer's work focused on defense mechanisms that can emerge through the art-making process, most notably that of sublimation (Kramer, 2001). *Sublimation* can be defined simply as the process of shifting emotional energies—which according to Freud, originate from sexual impulses (Erwin, 2002)—onto more socially constructive actions or behaviors. In art therapy, both the process and product, mutually, can serve as the outlet for which sublimation may occur. Rubin's (2008) film *Children & the Arts* illustrates how the process of sublimation can be achieved through any of the music, play, dance, drama, and art processes. Sublimation, Kramer (2001) asserts, can be cultivated but not forced, and not every process or product is evidence that this transformation has occurred.

Donald Winnicott, known for his contributions to object relations theory, has also influenced art therapy. Winnicott's (1971) theory of child development originates within the *transitional space*, or the area in between experiencing the differences of illusionary internal perceptions and outer reality, a process that begins during infancy. This process helps children develop the creative ability to place greater value on a particular item or object than the item itself, thus becoming the *transitional object*. The teddy bear and the baby blanket carried by children for security and soothing are prototypical examples. The artwork created in therapy, Malchiodi (2003) suggests, can assume the role of the *transitional object* by fulfilling the function of supportive therapist in his or her absence and serves as a reminder of what was learned in therapy.

McCullough (2009) describes how a child coping with divorce brought transitional objects from home early on in treatment; during the crux of therapy, they became the subject matter of the artwork, and their use diminished as the child was able to regain emotional constancy through the therapeutic relationship. The *transitional space* or, in therapy, the *holding environment* (Winnicott, 1971) is the therapeutic milieu where children can creatively repair deficient early object relations experiences through play and art-making. The role of the art therapist is that of facilitator of the creative environment, who is attuned to children's object relations, and that of a provider of supportive yet firm boundaries as children encounter pain resulting from unmet developmental experiences in order to facilitate growth, meaning, a sense of control, and healthy individuation (Robbins, 2001).

Developmental

Developmental art therapy emphasizes the comprehensive understanding of the normative process of cognitive, emotional, physical, and artistic development of children and the precept that creative artistic activities offer normative experiences and promote increased social, emotional, and cognitive functioning for all individuals (Malchiodi, Kim, & Choi, 2003; Rosal, 1992; Rubin, 1999, 2005; Uhlin & Chiaro, 1984; Williams & Wood, 1977). Art educator Viktor Lowenfeld contributed to this approach with his "art education therapy," which emphasized the use of creativity to foster the cognitive, emotional, and social growth of children (Lowenfeld & Brittain, 1987). Lowenfeld and Brittain's (1987) stages of normal artistic development in children provide a chronological framework for understanding graphic representations as an indicator of typical growth. Drawing from his seminal work, other theorists have contributed to an overall understanding of artistic development in children with similar chronologies (Gardner, 1994; Kellogg, 1970; Lansing, 1971; McFee, 1970). Art therapists possess a strong foundational knowledge of theories of normal artistic development in order to correctly identify atypical characteristics in child artwork, possible delays, or regression in development, and to provide interventions that best address the individual needs of children (Aach-Feldman & Kunkle-Miller, 2001; Anderson, 1992; Malchiodi et al., 2003).

Susan Aach-Feldman and Carole Kunkle-Miller (2001) integrate Piagetian cognitive theory in their developmental approach with children with severe cognitive, emotional, and physical disabilities. Children in Piaget's *Sensorimotor* phase of development (Piaget & Inhelder, 1966), typically between 0 and 2 years old, are involved in the process of understanding the world through sensory exploration, resulting in the understanding of self as other and simple cause-and-effect relationships. The developmental art therapist working with children in this phase might provide opportunities for them to practice movements used in art-making (grasping, touching, smearing), engage with materials that offer sensory stimulation (finger paints, foam, sand, clay), and model appropriate use of materials by playing with the children (Aach-Feldman & Kunkle-Miller, 2001). Children in the *Preoperational* phase, typically between 2 and 7 years old, marked by the children's ability to develop visual, motoric, and verbal symbols, begin to develop more logical and organized thinking (Piaget & Inhelder, 1966). Play and exploration of art materials are used with children in this phase to enhance their ability to discriminate concepts, encourage independent activity and confidence, and foster accurate identification of feeling states (Aach-Feldman & Kunkle-Miller, 2001). This approach is process oriented, whereby the objective is to nurture self-growth and skill acquisition through directed, playful, and sensorial engagement with the art materials.

Silver's (2001, 2002) contributions to art therapy emerged through her work with children with hearing impairments and her observation of them being inaptly labeled as cognitively impaired. This prompted her to construct several assessments used to evaluate and advance cognitive skills through art, and serve as an alternative to verbal tests of cognition. The development of her assessment tools and treatment interventions were influenced by multiple theorists, notably:

- Bruner's (1966) theoretical work, which posited cognition as a constructivist device for understanding the world
- Piaget and Inhelder's (1966) observations of logical thinking and ability to generalize prior to the development of language in children, and their experiments of conservation and classification
- Witkin's (1962) theory of psychological differentiation accounting for cognitive styles as dependent on different modes of thinking, including visual-spatial
- Arnheim's (2004) work, which supports the idea that visual perception, itself, is evidence of higher level cognitive processing

Silver (2001, 2002) posited that art therapy can help children (a) understand spatial concepts through representational drawing of objects, (b) learn to sequence through activities involving color theory and basic clay construction, (c) learn to group and categorize through her *stimulus drawings*, and (d) develop the ability to abstract through the process of selection and combination to form a new whole. The objective of the art therapist, according to Silver (2001), is to devise art interventions that provide opportunities for exploratory learning through hands-on tasks children find stimulating and rewarding and expand children's ability to communicate.

Adaptive art therapy theory primarily seeks to provide normalizing experiences for children with varying disabilities (Rosal, 1992). This key characteristic is interwoven, one might argue, within the framework of all art therapists, regardless of their theoretical stances. Anderson (1992) advocates that a child's ability, or disability, should not preclude participation in art activities and education. The onus is on the therapist to devise adaptations that ensure child participation and offer maximum benefit for all children. Adaptations may be applied to (a) the setting and surroundings, (b) the art mediums, (c) the instruments used to create, and (d) the methods of instruction (Anderson, 1992; Malchiodi et al., 2003). The therapist may store tools and materials on shelves that are at an accessible height for small children or those in a wheelchair. A cloth, or thin foam liner, can be wrapped around a pencil and taped in place for individuals who are in need of a better a grip. If a child with limited pincer grasp is creating a collage, the therapist may instruct the child to (1) hold a pencil in reverse; (2) select an item to be glued; (3) gently press the item with the eraser; and (4) press the eraser with the selected item attached onto the desired location precoated with glue.

The previous example, furthermore, serves as a narrative of task analysis. This technique may be used to break down an art activity into clear, concise, manageable steps that when sequenced together promote successful completion on behalf of children (Anderson, 1992). This may be augmented by the use of a graphic organizer, which pictorially depicts each step of the project; it can be created by the therapist or by children as a way to quickly document directions for use as a visual reference (Burau & Lombardi, 2011, 2012). Nonverbal students may use the picture exchange communication system (PECS), or an electronic version of the system, to communicate simple requests and needs such as, but not limited to, (a) the desire to work with paint, crayon, or pencil; (b) color choice; or (c) the need to wash their hands. The primary rationale for use of the aforementioned adaptations is the promotion of autonomous functioning, which in turn facilitates self-reliance and builds self-esteem.

Cognitive-Behavioral

Cognitive-behavioral therapy (CBT) draws from social learning (Rotter, 1982), behavioral (Skinner, 1976; Wolpe, 1958), cognitive (Beck, 1976), and social cognitive approaches (Bandura, 1986; D'Zurilla & Goldfried, 1971; Ellis, 2001; Kelly, 1963; Meichenbaum & Deffenbacher, 1988; Meichenbaum & Goodman, 1971; Mischel, 1996); it has strong evidence-based research documenting its efficacy in treatment. Ellis (2001), who was responsible for developing Rational Emotive Behavior Therapy (REBT), espoused the concept that thinking, feeling, and behaving are an interrelated cognitive process that can be either self-helping or self-destructive. When applied, the process of disputing irrational thoughts and beliefs is able to ameliorate negative feeling states and dysfunctional behavior, a tenet that is central to the CBT paradigm.

Kelly (1963) postulated that people use *personal* constructs, or ways of interpreting the world based on past experience, as predictors of future outcomes. In this theory, maladaptive emotional reactions occur when people do not have adequate constructs to understand a given experience. Meichenbaum and Goodman (1971) developed *self-instruction training* techniques to teach impulsive children to coach themselves through completion of motor tasks such as drawing and coloring. *Stress inoculation training*, a three-phase process, teaches clients to apply cognitive restructuring to their inner thoughts, dialogues, and mental imagery followed by experiential-based interventions, such as role-play and in-vivo desensitization (Wolpe, 1958), which provide children with graduated opportunities to practice learned skills (Meichenbaum & Deffenbacher, 1988). D'Zurilla and Goldfried (1971) employed problem-solving therapy, which uses task analysis to help clients (1) define the problem, (2) identify the desired result, (3) brainstorm possible solutions, (4) implement them, and (5) evaluate their effectiveness.

Marcia Rosal (1992, 1993, 2001; Rosal, McCulloch-Vislisel, Neece, 1997) brought attention to cognitive-behavioral art therapy in the field's literature. She and others have drawn from the psychological theories and interventions discussed previously in their applications with children. Rosal (2001) posits that children's artwork offers access to their mental imagery and personal construct system. This imagery, effused in the artwork, can then be used (a) to enable their understanding of their behavior (Epp, 2008; Henley, 1998; Rosal, 1992, 1993, 2001); (b) to identify and understand affect (Epp, 2008; Pifalo, 2007; Steele, 2003); (c) to generate solutions to problems (Henley, 1998; Pifalo, 2007; Rosal, 1992, 1993, 2001); (d) to increase self-awareness (Rosal, 1992); (e) to recognize cognitive distortions and mental messages (DeFrancisco, 1983; Rosal, 1992, 1993, 2001; Steele, 2003); (f) to promote change in behavior through cognitive restructuring (Epp, 2008; Rosal, 1992, 1993, 2001; Steele, 2003); (g) to increase coping skills with *stress inoculation* techniques (DeFrancisco, 1983; Pifalo, 2007; Rosal, 1992); (h) as the source of relaxation (Rosal, 1992); and (i) to increase the internal locus of control (Bowen & Rosal, 1989; Pifalo, 2007; Rosal, 1992, 1993, 2001; Steele, 2003). Art therapy complements and enhances existing applications of CBT. In the current paradigm of brief and solution-focused treatment, cognitive-behavioral art therapy offers a useful approach in a variety of settings.

The modality of art therapy was built without a concrete theory attached, and like a chameleon, it is able to morph and adapt inconspicuously to fit into a variety of theoretical models that are appropriate to serve the individual needs of clients. For example, a psychodynamic art therapy approach may not be appropriate for a 5-year-old child with autism who has limited receptive and expressive language skills, but an adaptive developmental art therapy approach may be suitable. This does not mean that art therapy is devoid of limitations in its theoretical approach, but its adaptability does help minimize them.

RESEARCH

Evidence-based practices are the substance of current mental health treatment models. Art therapy research suggests that it can be an effective modality for treating a variety of issues and circumstances of childhood and adolescence.

Pifalo (2006) evaluated the efficacy of a 60-minute, 8-week, trauma-focused cognitive-behavioral art therapy group with child victims of sexual abuse ($n = 41$). Comparison of participant pre- and post-assessment scores from the Trauma Symptom Checklist for Children (Briere, 1995, as cited in Pifalo, 2006) found statistically significant decreases among nine of ten subscales for posttrauma symptoms. In a separate randomized, controlled experimental study, Lyshak-Stelzer, Singer, St. John, and Chemtob (2007) examined the efficacy of a 60-minute, 16-week trauma-focused group art therapy intervention in decreasing posttrauma symptoms for adolescents ($n = 14$) as compared to a general activity-making control group ($n = 15$). Pre- and posttesting using the UCLA Post Traumatic Stress Disorder (PTSD) Reaction Index for DSM-IV, Child Version (Rodriguez, Steinberg, & Pynoos, 1999, as cited in Lyshak-Stelzer et al., 2007) found substantial statistically significant decreases of PTSD symptoms for children in the art therapy treatment group.

Hartz and Thick (2005) found that ten 90-minute art as therapy and art psychotherapy groups, when compared, were mutually beneficial for increasing self-esteem in adolescent female offenders ($n = 31$). Pre- and postintervention scores using the Harter Self-Perception Profile for Adolescents (Harter, 1988, as cited in Hartz & Thick, 2005) showed statistically significant increase in general social acceptance for participants of the art as therapy cohort, and significant increase in closer personal friendships for participants of the art psychotherapy group.

A study by Epp (2008) evaluated the effectiveness of a 60-minute, 9-month weekly group using art therapy with cognitive-behavioral strategies to develop social skills for children on the autism spectrum ($n = 66$). Pre- and posttest scores using the Social Skills Rating System (SSRS; Gresham & Elliot, 1990, as cited in Epp, 2008) completed by parents and educators of students revealed statistically significant increase in assertiveness, decrease of internalizing behaviors, decrease of hyperactivity, and an overall decrease of problematic behaviors for participants.

Favara-Scacco, Smirne, Schiliro, and Di Cataldo (2001) investigated the effectiveness of art therapy to decrease fear and anxiety during painful medical procedures associated with leukemia in children and adolescents ($n = 32$). They provided a systematic approach to treatment by using specific art therapy interventions prior to, during, and following medical procedures. Observed behavioral responses to treatment were used to evaluate efficacy. They noted that children who participated in the art therapy program coped more effectively and were more cooperative during the medical procedures. Poststudy, participants and their parents requested art therapy services when the procedures needed to be repeated, suggesting that participants perceived efficacy.

A major limitation in the field of art therapy is the limited amount of quantitative random, controlled experimental studies used to evaluate and substantiate the efficacy of the approach. There are, however, numerous qualitative, phenomenological, single case studies, single group without control group, and controlled nonrandomized research studies that buttress the practice. Slayton, D'Archer, and Kaplan (2010) suggest that those studies often use anecdotal information to validate treatment outcomes, do not always indicate specific treatment protocols for study replication, and at times mix art therapy with other treatment interventions, making it difficult to isolate treatment effect. In 2000, Reynolds, Nabors, and Quinlan completed a systematic review of the literature for empirical research on art therapy efficacy prior to 1999. They found only five randomized, controlled experimental studies. More recently, Slayton et al.'s (2010) identical review found 11 quantitative randomized, controlled studies published between 1999 and 2007. Their findings suggest that the profession is responding to remediate this limitation.

ART THERAPY: PROCESS AND PROCEDURES

The process or approaches to art therapy are as varied as there are theories of applied psychotherapy. The approaches used depend on myriad clinical details. Presenting problems, clinical diagnosis, chronological age, and stages of cognitive and emotional development will mutually impact the approach and interventions used in therapy. Treatment setting (educational environment, outpatient, inpatient medical, inpatient residential, community-based), length (single, brief, extended), and type (individual, group, family) will also delineate specific processes employed. The theoretical orientation of the art therapist will likely influence the ways in which he or she uses art therapy with clients.

Regardless of the process, all art therapists must consider specific procedures. The art therapy process, akin to other treatment modalities, begins with an intake session, including a needs assessment of the child. The art therapist may also elect to observe the child as she or he completes one or more art-based assessments to determine (a) the appropriateness of fit of the therapeutic modality and the client, (b) the types of art interventions and mediums the child may be most responsive or aversive toward (Kaplan, 2003), (c) the child's level of cognitive and emotional development (Anderson, 1992; Oster & Gould, 1987; Silver, 2002), and (d) the child's strengths and limitations (Kaplan, 2003; Oster & Gould, 1987). In the case of family art therapy, the therapist may use art-based assessment procedures to determine family dynamics, assigned roles, communication patterns, and perceived problems (Kwiatkowska, 1978; Landgarten, 1987).

Planning is an essential component of the art therapy session. The art therapist takes careful consideration of the client's treatment goals and objectives when planning art interventions (Silverstone, 2009). An essential question to ask oneself when creating an intervention is: What is the rationale for using this intervention, and which treatment objectives will the intervention address? The art therapist takes into account both the session length (30, 50, or 75 minutes) and time necessary to complete the art experience and process the artwork (Silverstone, 2009). Art therapists also consider to what degree they will interact with the client or facilitate the art materials throughout the session (Rubin, 1999, 2005). For example, if the therapist is concerned with assessment, he or she may occupy the role of observer. Or, if the therapist is concerned with deepening meaning for the client, the therapist may vacillate between the role of observer and that of educator or technical facilitator. Ensuring that one has the appropriate media required to complete a specific intervention or assessment is an essential aspect of the planning process. Art materials present in the art therapy room may include, but are not limited to, pencils, crayons, paints, pastels, papers (various sizes, textures, and colors), glues, scissors, chenille sticks, nonhardening modeling clay, nonhardening sticky foam, magazines, cardboard boxes, feathers, stickers, glitter glue, beads, string, wire, tapes, cameras, yarns, and fabrics.

Much clinical information can be obtained through the process of observation. The art therapist needs to be attuned to verbal, nonverbal, visual, and metaphorical methods of communication as indicators of clinical significance (Kaplan, 2003). Some of the questions art therapists might ask themselves include, but are not limited to, the following:

- In what manner did the child engage with the art materials?
- What media did the child select or decline?
- How much time did it take for the child to complete the art task?
- Did the child rush through or carefully attend to every detail of the art task?
- How much time was spent erasing and reworking?
- Was a final product achieved within the given time frame?
- Was the child able to use the art materials appropriately?
- Did the child paint over or cover up any images in the art? If so, what were they?
- What was the content and context, or lack thereof, of verbalizations that the child made while working?
- What type, frequency, and manner of nonverbal gestures, if any, were made?
- Were the gestures or verbalizations directed toward the art medium, self, or another participating party?

Information gleaned from these observations can provide insight into social, emotional, and cognitive development, frustration tolerance, personality characteristics, resistance, quality of self-talk, and media preferences of the child.

Upon completion of the art product, the art therapist might ask the child to describe the artwork via open-ended questions designed to clarify and facilitate understanding of the imagery created (Rubin, 2005). Examples of this type of inquiry might be, but are not limited to, the following:

- Please describe your artwork in as much detail as possible.
- If the person (animal, tree, building, car, object, color, line, etc.) in your artwork could speak, what would he/she/it say?
- If you could be any part of your artwork, what part would you be and why?
- Tell a story, with a beginning, middle, and end, about the people (animals, trucks, monsters, colors, objects, etc.) in your artwork.
- Write a list of all of the words that come to your mind when you look at your artwork.

Through this in-depth discussion about the child's imagery, the therapist gains an understanding of the child's symbolic language. It is important that the therapist not assign meaning to the content of image based on personal associations and projections—even in scenarios where the client is unable to verbalize the meaning of what was created. This approach helps ensure that the art therapist respects the multicultural differences of the client, as symbolic meanings vary depending on macro-, micro-, and meso-cultures (Bronfenbrenner, 1981).

The art therapist gives careful consideration to feedback provided, if any, on the art product. Creating an environment where children feel safe to experiment, explore, and play is of utmost importance, because that is where learning and growth can happen. Feedback that contains appraisal or judgment occludes therapeutic rapport, whereas empathic response toward and precise observations of created artwork supports the alliance. Value is placed on the process and the information delivered therein, rather than only on the end product.

PRACTICAL TECHNIQUES

The techniques and interventions used by art therapists are usually simple prompts for children to engage with the art media. Prompts can be directive, "Draw what sad looks like to you," or nondirective, "Draw, paint, color a subject of your choice." Although interventions to address specific problems exist, art therapists are just as likely to create and adapt art interventions to address the needs of the moment. The case illustration provides examples of five interventions. Many of the interventions can be adapted to address treatment issues or scenarios other than those presented in the illustration. Possibilities for potential adaptions are also provided.

Case Study

Sarah is a soft-spoken and shy 15-year-old girl with long brown hair. Her father initiated counseling services for her, her brother, Ben, and himself after having been in a near-fatal automobile accident. They had been driving around dusk when a speeding vehicle ran a red light and crashed into their small-sized sport utility vehicle. The vehicle flipped and rolled several times before sliding on its roof into the grassy area alongside the highway intersection. The family, unable to open the locked doors of the vehicle, was trapped. Good Samaritans broke out the windows and pulled the family out prior to emergency medical team arrival. The family reported that within minutes of being pulled from the wreckage, they witnessed their vehicle explode. They were all taken by ambulance to the hospital to be evaluated. Ben suffered a mild concussion, the father required multiple surgeries, and Sarah experienced hematomas and minor lacerations on various parts of her body.

At school, Sarah received attention from staff and students, who were curious to know more about the accident and how she was coping. Extended family members did the same. The continuous inquiries contributed to high levels of anxiety and, at times, panic for Sarah. She reported perceiving that she was reliving the accident "over and over again," whenever someone probed about the experience, and she wanted people to stop inquiring about the accident. She reported physiological symptoms such as (a) difficulties sleeping, including nightmares about the explosion, (b) racing heart rate, (c) accelerated breathing, (d) body sweats, and (e) an inability to stop crying. She also reported experiencing the same symptoms immediately following loud noises and sirens from fire trucks, ambulances, and police vehicles. Perhaps most significant was her fear of riding in the car. She reported that she had been spending the duration of car rides tense and tearful.

During the second meeting with Sarah, she completed a projective bridge drawing (Figure 3.1). She was asked to "Draw a bridge that connects your life before and after the accident." This initial drawing was

Figure 3.1   Sarah's First Bridge

completed over two sessions. Sarah worked in a very slow and deliberate fashion as she created each element of the bridge drawing. She took time to sit and contemplate her image prior to making marks on the paper. The image, long and linear, appears flattened and drawn from an aerial perspective—looking down at the bridge from above. The perspective used in the drawing is representative of Lowenfeld's Schematic stage of development (Lowenfeld & Brittain, 1987), typically occurring between ages 7 and 9, so it is an indicator of a possible developmental regression as a result of the trauma and her current need to view the experience from a distance. She wrote the words "before" and "after" over each side and used rectangles of color on each side to represent her affective state. The "before" side had large swatches of pink and purple, which represented her feeling happy and fun-loving, and a small swatch of blue, which represented feelings of sadness. On the "after" side, she placed a large rectangle of blue to represent sadness, reflective of her inability to stop crying and regulate her emotions. The rain clouds under the bridge represent the "storm" of the accident.

In the initial stage of treatment, Sarah created a destress ball. The ball was created by: (1) inserting a balloon inside another of the same size, (2) inserting dried beans, sand, or rice into the balloon opening until it was full enough to experience resistance when squeezed, and

(3) tying it off and decorating it. Sarah cloaked her destress ball with fabric to protect it from being punctured. The destress ball was used to teach deep-breathing and deep-muscle relaxation exercises through squeezing and releasing the ball in sync with breathwork. It served as a transitional object, a physical reminder to use the practiced relaxation techniques, during stressful commutes in the car.

Sarah was asked to "Create an image, using magazine photos, of what your anxiety looks like." She assembled a large cactus covered with long, prickly needles in the center of a desert landscape. Guided imagery exercises, based on her cactus metaphor, were practiced to make the anxiety more manageable. Sarah suggested creating a guided imagery exercise with the cactus jumping rope and another as a rocket shooting off into outer space. The juxtaposition of the spiny cactus jumping rope or as a rocket made her laugh out loud, thus creating an affective shift, which minimized the fear and stress associated with the anxiety.

Once she was equipped with a few anxiety management techniques, Sarah was instructed to "Use a pencil to draw a time-sequenced narrative of your day beginning several hours prior to, during, and several hours after the accident." She was given a piece of paper with several small rectangles framed by black lines, to provide containment, to complete the drawings. The intervention was completed over the course of multiple sessions—a slow, safe progressive reexposure to the trauma to avoid hyperarousal and emotional flooding. Sarah set the pace of the narrative. During creation and discussion of each image, Sarah was asked to identify her sensory experiences (e.g., sights, smells, breathing patterns, heart rate, increased body temperature or sweats) and any self-talk associated with the specific aspect of the narrative. Cognitive reframing techniques were used to counteract maladaptive thought patterns that emerged as a result of the trauma. Sarah used the destress ball coupled with relaxation and guided imagery techniques immediately following the reexperiencing procedure, as a closing method to the therapy sessions. The reexperiencing process was repeated until Sarah was able to tolerate reviewing the entire event, including her thoughts, feelings, and memories, without significant emotional distress.

Toward the close of sessions, Sarah completed another projective bridge drawing (Figure 3.2) using the same instructions as the first.

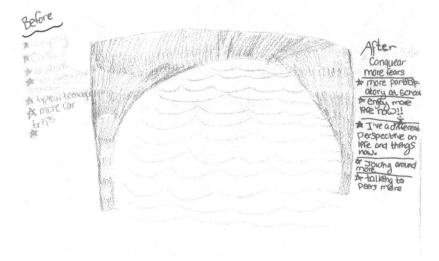

Before

After
Conquear
more fears
★ more particip-
atory at school
★ enjoy more
free roam!!
★ I've a different
perspective on
life and things
now.
★ joking around
more
★ talking to
peers more

Figure 3.2   Sarah's Second Bridge

She quickly began to sketch and color in the physical structure of the bridge. She created the image and the lists of words accompanying the drawing without hesitation. This bridge appears three-dimensional, unlike the flattened structure she created prior to treatment. Under the bridge she added water and reported that this represented "life." As in the initial drawing, she added the titles "before" and "after" on each side of the bridge, but this time she listed words and phrases she associated with both. Notably, phrases on the "after" side focused on the positive aspects of her behavioral and affective functioning, rather than her prior emotional state of just sadness. The perspective of the final drawing is representative of Lowenfeld's pseudo-naturalistic stage of artistic development (Lowenfeld & Brittain, 1987), one closer to her actual chronological age, and an indicator that the regression apparent in the original drawing had been resolved, or that she now had the ability to tolerate viewing the event.

In the second-to-last session, Sarah completed her final image in art therapy. She was asked to "Create, using any of the art materials available in the therapy room, an image of *what you need* as you transition out of therapy." Sarah selected several rolls of colored tape and affixed large strips of yellow tape in a woven pattern onto the paper and wrote the word "supported" (Figure 3.3).

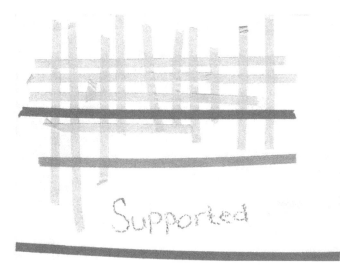

Figure 3.3   Sarah's Final Art Project: Support

She discussed the many ways in which she experienced feeling supported by a tightly woven network of family, friends, teachers, and
administrators at school, and by a therapist through the process of learning to cope after the traumatic accident. This represented an important
shift in Sarah's perceptive experience. Upon intake she was unable to
take in the support being offered by her social network, because she
experienced their inquiries as a trigger for her posttrauma symptoms. She
articulated that she was ready to end therapy, because she believed she
would continue to feel "supported" in her daily life.

Sarah's case illustrates the use of five art therapy interventions in the
treatment of an adolescent with posttrauma symptoms:

- The pre- and postintervention bridge drawing provided a comparative assessment of the child's perception of current functioning
  and progress made in therapy. The intervention can be adapted
  for a variety of presenting problems by replacing the word "accident" in the directive with another life transition, such as, but
  not limited to, abuse, divorce, illness, or loss.
- The creation of the destress ball and concurrent use with relaxation techniques helped Sarah generalize skills learned in therapy
  into her daily routine.

- Through a simple collage made of magazine photo images, Sarah was able to communicate her total-body experience of anxiety. Guided imagery exercises were tailored to her visual metaphors and implemented to promote affective change when she was experiencing anxiety. This exercise can be adapted to media (draw, paint, sculpt) and to emotions (fear, anger, sadness) to assist clients in gaining mastery over their affective experience.

- The trauma narrative intervention allowed Sarah to reexperience the trauma at her own pace, promoting a sense of safety and control over the experience. The use of pencil, not fluid or noneraseable media, and drawing within the small, framed rectangles also helped facilitate a sense of control and containment for Sarah. The ritual of ending the session with the relaxation techniques was twofold: (1) It served as a practice of relaxation techniques to promote mastery of skills, and (2) it served as a method of emotional reintegration and closure from the traumatic material.

- The *what you need* picture, used as a termination exercise with Sarah, can be adapted, but is not limited, to treatment plan development, exploration of familial relationships, or the experience of success as a learner. Responding to the question of "what one needs" can help clients to develop intrapersonal insight and awareness and generate solutions to problems. In the case of Sarah, it demonstrated the successful cognitive restructuring of her experience and her readiness to terminate treatment.

CONCLUSION

This chapter provides a general overview of some of the theories and applications that inform the practice of art therapy. The information provided should not be considered comprehensive. The history of the profession is as rich, colorful, and dynamic as the practice itself. It draws from the work of many influential psychological and educational theorists across paradigms. Applications of art therapy can assimilate to multiple theoretical models, sometimes at the same time, thus promoting individualized and appropriate treatment methods. As such, art therapy can be an effective modality for treating a variety of issues that present in childhood and adolescence. Perhaps the greatest rationale for using art in therapy with children is that, akin to play, children use art as a natural method for understanding their world.

SPECIALIZED TRAINING AND RESOURCES

Associations

The American Art Therapy Association (AATA)
4875 Eisenhower Avenue, Suite 240
Alexandria, VA 22304
www.arttherapy.org

The Art Therapy Credentials Board (ATCB)
3 Terrace Way
Greensboro, NC 27403-3660
1-877-213-2822
www.atcb.org

National Coalition of Creative Arts Therapies Associations (NCCATA)
www.nccata.org

International Expressive Arts Therapies Association (IEATA)
P.O. Box 320399
San Francisco, CA 94132
415-522-8959
www.ieata.org

Educational Requirements

A Master's degree in art therapy, which includes 48 credit hours of graduate-level coursework in content areas of art therapy and counseling, is required for practice.

The Art Therapy Credentials Board (ATCB) is the credentialing body for art therapy practitioners. Registered Art Therapist (ATR) requires completion of a Master's-level education program and post-graduate supervised clinical experience. Board Certification (ATR-BC) requires completion of the ATR requirements and successfully passing the Art Therapy Credentials Board Exam (ATCBE). The Art Therapy Credentialed Supervisor (ATCS) requires an ATR-BC and demonstration of competence in art therapy supervision.

Conferences and Trainings

- The AATA Conference is hosted annually within the United States. For more information visit www.arttherapy.org
- The Institute for Continuing Education in Art Therapy (ICE/AT) offers continuing education credits, as an approved provider for the National Board for Certified Counselors (NBCC), via online classes. For more information, visit http://arttherapy.train ingcampus.net
- The Expressive Therapies Summit, sponsored by Expressive Media, Inc., is an annual interdisciplinary arts therapies conference held each November in New York City. For more information, visit www.expressivetherapiessummit.com
- The IEATA Conference is an expressive arts therapies conference hosted in a different international location every 2 years. For more information, visit www.ieata.org/conference.html

Audiovisual Materials

Expressive Media, Inc. produces and distributes numerous DVDs about the expressive arts therapies. For more information, visit www .expressivemedia.org.

REFERENCES

Aach-Feldman, S., & Kunkle-Miller, C. (2001). Developmental art therapy. In J. Rubin (Ed.), *Approaches to art therapy: Theory & technique* (2nd ed., pp. 226–240). Philadelphia, PA: Brunner-Routledge.

American Art Therapy Association. (2012). *About us: History of art therapy.* Retrieved from http://www.americanarttherapyassociation.org/aata-history -background.html

Anderson, F. E. (1992). *Art for all the children: Approaches to art therapy for children with disabilities* (2nd ed.). Springfield, IL: Charles C. Thomas.

Arnheim, R. (2004). *Visual thinking: Thirty-fifth anniversary printing.* Berkeley: University of California Press.

Bandura, A. (1986). *Social foundations of thought and action: A social cognitive theory.* Englewood Cliffs, NJ: Prentice-Hall.

Beck, A. T. (1976). *Cognitive therapy and the emotional disorders.* New York, NY: International Universities Press.

Beveridge, A. (2001). A disquieting feeling of strangeness?: The art of the mentally ill. *Journal of the Royal Society of Medicine, 94*(11), 595–599.

Bowen, C. A., & Rosal, M. L. (1989). The use of art therapy to reduce the maladaptive behaviors of a mentally retarded adult. *The Arts in Psychotherapy, 16,* 211–218.

Bronfenbrenner, U. (1981). *The ecology of human development: Experiments by nature and design.* Cambridge, MA: Harvard University Press.

Bruner, J. S. (1966). *Studies in cognitive growth.* New York, NY: Wiley.

Burau, D. E., & Lombardi, R. L. (2011). *Art therapy for children with autism in educational settings.* Paper presented at the Second Annual Expressive Therapies Summit, New York, NY.

Burau, D. E., & Lombardi, R. L. (2012). *Intertwining art therapy and education for special needs children.* Advanced Practice Course presented at the 43rd Annual Conference of the American Art Therapy Association, Savannah, GA.

Cane, F. (1983). *The artist in each of us.* Craftsbury Common, VT: Art Therapy Publications.

DeFrancisco, J. (1983). Implosive art therapy: A learning-theory based psychodynamic approach. In L. Gantt & S. Whitman (Eds.), *Proceedings of the Eleventh Annual Conference of the American Art Therapy Association* (pp. 74–79). Baltimore, MD: American Art Therapy Association.

D' Zurilla, T. J., & Goldfried, M. R. (1971). Problem solving and behavior modification. *Journal of Abnormal Psychology, 78,* 107–126.

Edwards, D. (2004). Art therapy. In P. Wilkins (Series Ed.), *Creative therapies in practice.* London, England: Sage.

Ellis, A. (2001). *Overcoming destructive beliefs, feelings, and behaviors: New directions for rational emotive behavior therapy.* Amherst, NY: Prometheus.

Epp, K. M. (2008). Outcome-based evaluation of a social skills program using art therapy and group therapy for children on the autism spectrum. *Children & Schools*, 30(1), 27–36.

Erwin, E. (Ed.). (2002). *The Freud encyclopedia: Theory, therapy, and culture*. New York, NY: Routledge.

Favara-Scacco, D., Smirne, G., Schiliro, G., & Di Cataldo, A. (2001). Art therapy as support for children with leukemia during painful procedures. *Medical Pediatric Oncology*, 36(4), 478–480.

Gardner, H. (1994). *The arts and human development*. New York, NY: Basic Books.

Hartz, L., & Thick, L. (2005). Art therapy strategies to raise self-esteem in female juvenile offenders: A comparison of art psychotherapy and art as therapy approaches. *Art Therapy: Journal of the American Art Therapy Association*, 22(2), 70–80.

Henley, D. (1998). Art therapy in a socialization program for children with attention deficit hyperactivity disorder. *American Journal of Art Therapy*, 37(1), 2–12.

Hogan, S. (2001). *Healing arts: The history of art therapy*. London, England: Jessica Kingsley.

Junge, M. B. (2010). *The modern history of art therapy in the United States*. Springfield, IL: Charles C. Thomas.

Kaplan, F. (2003). Art-based assessments. In C. A. Malchiodi (Ed.), *Handbook of art therapy* (pp. 25–35). New York, NY: Guilford Press.

Kellogg, R. (1970). *Analyzing children's art*. Palo Alto, CA: Mayfield.

Kelly, G. A. (1963). *A theory of personality: The psychology of personal constructs*. New York, NY: W. W. Norton.

Kramer, E. (2000). A history and lineage of art therapy as practiced by Edith Kramer. In L. A. Gerity (Ed.), *Art as therapy: Collected papers* (pp. 20–25). London, England: Jessica Kingsley.

Kramer, E. (2001). Sublimation and art therapy. In J. Rubin (Ed.), *Approaches to art therapy: Theory & technique* (2nd ed., pp. 28–39). Philadelphia, PA: Brunner-Routledge.

Kwiatkowska, H. Y. (1978). *Family therapy and evaluation through art*. Springfield, IL: Charles C. Thomas.

Landgarten, H. B. (1987). *Family art psychotherapy: A clinical guide and casebook*. Levittown, PA: Brunner/Mazel.

Lansing, K. M. (1971). *Art, artists, and art education*. New York, NY: McGraw-Hill.

Leroi-Gourhan, A. (1982). The archaeology of Lascaux cave. *Scientific American*, 246(6), 104–112.

Lowenfeld, V., & Brittain, W. L. (1987). *Creative and mental growth* (8th ed.). Upper Saddle River, NJ: Prentice Hall.

Lyshak-Stelzer, F., Singer, P., St. John, P., & Chemtob, C. M. (2007). Art therapy for adolescents with posttraumatic stress disorder symptoms: A pilot study. *Art Therapy: Journal of the American Art Therapy Association, 24*(4), 163–169.

Malchiodi, C. A. (2003). Psychoanalytic, analytic, and object relations approaches. In C. A. Malchiodi (Ed.), *Handbook of art therapy* (pp. 41–57). New York, NY: Guilford Press.

Malchiodi, C. A., Kim, D. Y., & Choi, W. S. (2003). Developmental art therapy. In C. A. Malchiodi (Ed.), *Handbook of art therapy* (pp. 93–105). New York, NY: Guilford Press.

McFee, J. K. (1970). *Preparation for art.* Belmont, CA: Wadsworth.

Meichenbaum, D. H., & Deffenbacher, J. L. (1988). Stress inoculation training. *The Counseling Psychologist, 16*(1), 69–90.

Meichenbaum, D. H., & Goodman, J. (1971). Training impulsive children to talk to themselves: A means of developing self-control. *Journal of Abnormal Psychology, 77*, 115–126.

McCullough, C. (2009). A child's use of transitional objects in art therapy to cope with divorce. *Art Therapy: Journal of the American Art Therapy Association, 26*(1), 19–25.

Mischel, W. (1996). *Personality and assessment.* Mahwah, NJ: Lawrence Erlbaum.

Naumburg, M. (1987). *Dynamically oriented art therapy: Its principles and practices.* Chicago, IL: Magnolia Street.

Oster, G. D., & Gould, P. (1987). *Using drawings in assessment and therapy: A guide for mental health professionals.* New York, NY: Brunner-Routledge.

Piaget, J., & Inhelder, B. (1966). *The psychology of the child* (H. Weaver, Trans.). New York, NY: Basic Books.

Pifalo, T. (2006). Art therapy with sexually abused children and adolescents: Extended research study. *Art Therapy: Journal of the American Art Therapy Association, 23*(4), 181–185.

Pifalo, T. (2007). Jogging the cogs: Trauma-focused art therapy and cognitive behavioral therapy with sexually abused children. *Art Therapy: Journal of the American Art Therapy Association, 24*(4), 170–175.

Prinzhorn, H. (1972). *Artistry of the mentally ill* (E. von Brockdorff, Trans.). New York, NY: Springer-Verlag. [Originally published in 1922 as *Bildnerei der Geisteskanken*, Berlin: Verlag Julius Springer]

Reynolds, M. W., Nabors, L., & Quinlan, A. (2000). The effectiveness of art therapy: Does it work? *Art Therapy: Journal of the American Art Therapy Association, 17*(3), 207–213.

Robbins, A. (2001). Object relations and art therapy. In J. Rubin (Ed.), *Approaches to art therapy: Theory & technique* (2nd ed., pp. 54–65). Philadelphia, PA: Brunner-Routledge.

Rosal, M. L. (1992). Approaches to art therapy with children. In F. E. Anderson (Ed.), *Art for all the children* (pp. 142–183). Springfield, IL: Charles C. Thomas.

Rosal, M. L. (1993). Comparitive group art therapy research to evaluate changes in locus of control in behavior disordered children. *The Arts in Psychotherapy, 20,* 231–241.

Rosal, M. L. (2001). Cognitive-behavioral art therapy. In J. Rubin (Ed.), *Approaches to art therapy: Theory & technique* (2nd ed., pp. 210–225). Philadelphia, PA: Brunner-Routledge.

Rosal, M. L., McCulloch-Vislisel, S., & Neece, S. (1997). Keeping students in school: An art therapy approach to benefit ninth-grade students. *Art Therapy: Journal of the American Art Therapy Association, 14,* 30–36.

Rotter, J. B. (1982). *The development and application of social learning theory: Selected papers.* New York, NY: Praeger.

Rubin, J. A. (1999). *Art therapy: An introduction.* Philadelphia, PA: Brunner/Mazel.

Rubin, J. A. (2001a). Discovery, insight, and art therapy. In J. Rubin (Ed.), *Approaches to art therapy: Theory & technique* (2nd ed., pp. 15–27). Philadelphia, PA: Brunner-Routledge.

Rubin, J. A. (Ed.). (2001b). *Approaches to art therapy: Theory & technique* (2nd ed.). Philadelphia, PA: Brunner-Routledge.

Rubin, J. A. (2005). *Child art therapy* (25th anniversary edition). Hoboken, NJ: Wiley.

Rubin, J. A., & Expressive Media, Inc. (Producers). (2008). *The arts as therapy with children: Children & the arts* [DVD]. Available from www.expressivemedia .org/films.html

Sander, D. F., & Wong, S. H. (Eds.). (1997). *The sacred heritage: The influence of shamanism on analytical psychology.* New York, NY: Routledge.

Silver, R. (2001). Assessing and developing cognitive skills through art. In J. Rubin (Ed.), *Approaches to art therapy: Theory & technique* (2nd ed., pp. 241–253). Philadelphia, PA: Brunner-Routledge.

Silver, R. (2002). *Three art assessments: The silver drawing test of cognition and emotion; draw a story: screening for depression; and stimulus drawing and techniques.* New York, NY: Brunner-Routledge.

Silverstone, L. (2009). *Art therapy exercises: Inspirational and practical ideas to stimulate the imagination.* London, England: Jessica Kingsley.

Skinner, B. F. (1976). *About behaviorism.* New York, NY: Random House.

Slayton, S. C., D'Archer, J., & Kaplan, F. (2010). Outcome studies on the efficacy of art therapy: A review of the findings. *Art Therapy: Journal of the American Art Therapy Association, 27*(3), 108–119.

Steele, W. (2003). Using drawing in short-term trauma resolution. In C. A. Malchiodi (Ed.), *Handbook of art therapy* (pp. 139–151). New York, NY: Guilford Press.

Uhlin, D. M., & Chiaro, E. D. (1984). *Art for exceptional children* (3rd ed.). Dubuque, IA: William C. Brown.

Williams, G. H., & Wood, M. M. (1977). *Developmental art therapy.* Baltimore, MD: University Park Press.

Winnicott, D. W. (1971). *Playing and reality.* London, England: Tavistock/ Routledge.

Witkin, H. A. (1962). *Psychological differentiation: Studies of development.* New York, NY: Wiley.

Wolpe, J. (1958). *Psychotherapy by reciprocal inhibition.* Stanford, CA: Stanford University Press.

Drama Therapy

ELEANOR IRWIN

INTRODUCTION

Anyone watching a child playing at home, at school, or in a therapy room has probably marveled at the exuberance of the young player with a wild imagination and a storehouse of strange fantasies. Similarly, when enjoying the theatre or a movie, one can also admire the imagination of the playwright or screenwriter, wondering just where those crazy ideas came from! To therapists, however, the answer is easy. There have always been thorny disagreements about fantasy, play, and therapy, in general, but there is broad agreement that "those crazy ideas" come from the individual's early life experiences, which have a profound effect on one's future life.

As grown-ups, we tend to repress "crazy ideas," but nevertheless, these troubling thoughts and feelings sometimes find their way unwittingly into our everyday lives in dreams, slips of the tongue, or, more ominously, as physical or emotional symptoms of one kind or another. Theatre, like child's play, gives us temporary respite from past and present stress and troubling preoccupations. The "as if" stance of drama can provide relief from inner turmoil, because the activity affords intense, raw pleasure in playing things out, in pretending to be someone else, in doing something "foreign" to the self, while safely expressing the disguised guilty secrets in one's life.

The wish to play things out, whether in spontaneous drama or as an actor in the theatre, is part of the fascination of this art form, which is the basis for a discipline that is called Drama Therapy. Charles Durning, the well-known actor, articulately spoke to the core of the "as if" drama experience, which is universal:

> There are many secrets in us, in the depths of our souls that we don't want anyone else to know about. There's terror and repulsion in us, the terrible spot we don't talk about. That place that no one knows about. . . . A lot of that is released through acting. (Durning, 2012)

Drama and theatre have the power to expose the inner self, much as we try to repress "forbidden" thoughts and feelings in our attempts to hide them and to look "normal." For all of us, managing the tension between the inner, hidden self and the outer, visible self becomes more complicated as we move from childhood into adulthood. If development is on course, and with healthy genetic endowment (important considerations!), children's futures rest largely on an attuned relationship with a "good-enough" mother and a facilitating environment (Winnicott, 1965). Over time, if there is a secure attachment and smooth interaction between children and the environment, they forge healthy identifications with significant people in their lives.

As children mature, they begin to play out what they have seen, felt, dreamed, and fantasized, with actions and thoughts elaborated through roles, dialogue, and plot. Whether the play is about parents and babies, or devils and dinosaurs, the themes reflect what children or adolescents/adults are thinking, feeling, and/or fearing. So natural is this activity that Piaget considered play to be "a mirror for the ego," an aspect of the sensorimotor level of intelligence (Piaget, 1962). This kind of spontaneous play, rooted in early experience, is tapped in drama therapy, regardless of the age of the player.

DRAMA THERAPY: PROCESS AND PROCEDURES

Play Therapy: Precursor of Improvisational Drama

Soon after the birth of psychoanalysis in Vienna, child analysts, following the example of Sigmund Freud, noted the importance of children
as *individuals* rather than as *little adults*, which was a common misun-
derstanding of the day. Hearing about the anxiety of "Little Hans,"
who had a phobia about horses, Freud took pity on the child and, in
an effort to help him, encouraged the boy's father to treat him, under
Freud's supervision (Freud, 1955/1909). This successful experience
was significant, because it gave full recognition to the mental life of
children, and also acknowledged that "symptoms" (such as phobias)
have meanings that can be understood and resolved, even with little
children.

Work with Little Hans broadened the scope of psychoanalysis, paving
the way for child therapy. Individuals like Hermine von Hug-Hellmuth
(1921), credited with being the first analytic play therapist, Melanie
Klein (1932), Berta Bornstein (1949), and Joyce McDougall and Serge
Lobovici (1969), to mention just a few analysts, began to expand their
understanding and uses of play with neurotic as well as psychotic children. Their publications spread the word that children's "pretend" stories
and dramatizations were rooted in their unconscious, and that their deep
meanings could be tapped and utilized in therapy. Such enactments were
what Waelder (1933) called children's "partly digested" past and present
experiences, often attempts to turn from being passive victims to being
active participants—a wish to be the master of a confusing or traumatic
situation (Freud, 1955/1920). The following example, taken from early
work in drama therapy with children who had multiple operations for
cleft lip and palate (Irwin & McWilliams, 1974), illustrates Waelder's
principle of turning passive into active, Freud's explanation of play as an
attempt at mastery, and Bettelheim's (1987) belief that play is the royal
road to the unconscious.

A group of 4- and 5-year-old boys and girls relished the spontaneous playing out of stories of doctors and operations. Making masks for
themselves and their "patients," the doctors stretched out their peers

on chairs, and took turns operating on them, beginning many procedures with the stern comment, "You're *not* gonna die! Stay still!" Paradoxically, at the end of the operation, as the patient tried to find his way home, the "mother" refused him entrance, saying: "You're not MY boy—go away!"

In these vignettes, the children tried on the roles of doctor, patient, and mother, trying to see what it was like from another's point of view. Surely this was an attempt at mastery of a frightening, overwhelming situation and, as Waelder wrote, the attempt to turn from being passive "victims" (patients) to active "aggressors" (doctors). In addition, these preschoolers also tried to reassure themselves that death was *not* imminent ("You're *not* gonna die!"), while revealing their unconscious worries that the changes wrought by the operations would lead to further rejection from their loved ones.

Other Influences on Drama Therapy: Psychodrama, Gestalt, and Theatre

Even though there was no national organization or registration procedure for the field, early on I called my work Drama Therapy, adopting a name that emulated the other expressive arts therapies. Many other individuals in different parts of the country did the same, each looking for a framework that would give meaning and understanding to improvised drama or theatre experiences. Many also sought training in other action-oriented approaches, like Moreno's psychodrama, role play, and sociodrama (Moreno, 1946/1959/1962); Perls' Gestalt therapy (1969); Viola Spolin's (1975) theatre games; and the writings and work of Stanislavski (1936) and Grotowski (1965), among others.

It soon became clear to me as well as to others that more in-depth psychological training was necessary to understand the clinically rich material that emerged from the play of children and from the Spolin-based activities with adolescents and adults. We were well prepared in the drama/theatre component of the work, but we were less prepared for the therapy part of our still-new discipline. The need for further training was implied in Erikson's comment (1950, p. 222) about the core value of play:

> Modern play therapy is based on the observation that a child
> made insecure by a secret hate . . . seems able to use the pro-
> tective sanction of an understanding adult to regain some play
> peace. . . . For to "play it out" is the most natural self-healing
> measure childhood affords.

What became clear over time was that the "understanding adult" who
could help someone with a "secret hate" would also need in-depth therapeutic training.

Drama therapists have diverse training backgrounds, some in counseling, psychology, special education, social work, or educational or
therapeutic theatre. My background was in psychology, with advanced
training in psychoanalysis with children and adults, as well as in psychodrama and group therapy. Like many other beginning drama therapists,
I worked with those with disabilities—neurological, sensory, emotional,
and/or those with clefts of the lip and/or palate—and also worked col-
laboratively with other expressive arts therapists. Over time, these
experiences convinced me that in addition to pleasure and support,
improvisational drama also afforded an intimate look into the psychological lives of troubled children and their earnest efforts to overcome
their hidden psychic pain. The following description is an example of
one child's use of drama therapy as he participated in a group with other
emotionally disturbed children.

Many years ago, as a beginning drama therapist, I unknowingly
became one of Erikson's "understanding adults" working with a child
full of "secret hate," searching for "play peace." In an unusual program
at a Child Guidance Center, I worked with a group of emotionally disturbed, "acting-out" latency children, meeting for 6 hours per week over
a 3-month period. I was supervised by Marvin Shapiro, M.D., an analyst
and a lover of the arts, who was interested in knowing if and how drama
could be helpful with a difficult-to-reach population.

Jeremy, an FLK ("funny-looking kid"), full of squiggles, strange
speech, and even stranger behavior, was an isolate in the group, one
whom other group members could not understand. Retreating to a "safe
house" under a table, Jeremy began to periodically join the group by
darting out from his hideout. He either circled the group or ran smack

through the center of the circle, sometimes pantomiming or yelling that he was shooting with "live ammunition" and other times shouting that he was shooting them with a camera.

Stunned at first, the group members eventually became amused by Jeremy's wild imagination, and their growing attention to his fantasies allowed him, over time, to gradually begin to make a place for himself *in* the group, rather than as an *outside invader* of the group. In time, Jeremy's "crazy ideas" exuded a kind of contagion, and he became the leader of "the wild ones." Others, captivated, joined him in his forays, in fantasies that reflected his core anxieties of oral aggression, merger, abandonment, and/or death. Although I was unaware of it at the time, I later understood that Jeremy's play was something akin to primary process thinking, with images shifting constantly as in a dream, with displacement and condensation of scenes, themes, and roles. Slowly, and over time, Jeremy's wildness became less bizarre, easier to follow, often softened by his offbeat humor. By the end of the group he was the leader, not the follower, and the FLK designation faded into oblivion.

BLENDING DRAMA/THEATRE AND THERAPY IN NADTA

A smattering of articles and presentations at major conferences in the mid-1970s led a small group of practitioners to meet and talk, comparing backgrounds, styles of practice, and theoretical orientations. It soon became apparent that all of us had the same ultimate goal: the wish to use drama/theatre techniques to help relieve the psychological suffering of troubled individuals in their struggles to be more in control of their emotional lives.

In 1979, a few years after the formation of the Association for Dramatherapists in Great Britain, our own group, the National Association for Drama Therapy (NADT), came into being. Since that time, the organization has grown steadily, and in 2012, it officially changed its name to the North American Drama Therapy Association (NADTA) in recognition of the many drama therapists practicing throughout North America, especially in Canada. Like art, music, and movement/dance therapists, drama therapists work with people of all ages and disabilities, in diverse settings, from schools, prisons, and hospitals to clinics and community settings.

However, like our colleagues in other fields, we also have different ideas about the definition and training requirements of our field. Some drama therapists are theatre-oriented, whereas others work in an improvisational play style. Many different theoretical orientations and training backgrounds are represented in this group, including psychodrama and sociodrama; Maslow and Rogerian humanistic approaches; and different psychodynamic models, including those of Freud, Jung, and Perls, among others.

Although drama therapists wove a tapestry of many different colors, there was the early recognition that the NADT umbrella was large enough to encompass these divergent styles and modes of working, as is the case in the other expressive therapy fields. Over the years, the field has expanded and now includes those with many different therapeutic frameworks, including cognitive-behavioral therapy, shamanism, educational and/or therapeutic theatre, playback theatre, narrative, and storytelling. Similarly, the populations with whom drama therapists work has also broadened, encompassing people of all disabilities and ages, including newborns, autistic and psychotic individuals, as well as geriatric populations.

In 1982, Robert Landy offered a thorough review of the growing field in his article, "Training the Drama Therapist—A Four-Part Model" (Landy, 1982). In this seminal piece, Landy outlined the diverse backgrounds and appropriate training of drama therapists and suggested a training program that would (a) emphasize development of the self (which he called personal creativity and psychological awareness); (b) enhance understanding of those with disabilities; (c) provide training in drama/theatre and psychotherapy, supported by the study of drama therapy theory; and, (d) help establish supervised internships. Landy also pointed out many potential pitfalls in this discipline, citing a need for more research. For those interested in the field, his cogent and still-timely article is a must-read even though it was written in the early 1980s.

Similarly, an attempt to illustrate the wide diversity of the work by experienced drama therapists was undertaken by David Johnson and Penny Lewis in 2003 in *Approaches to Drama Therapy* (revised in 2009 by Johnson and Renee Emunah). This impressive overview covers contributions from experienced drama therapists who work in many different ways with people of all ages and disabilities. Johnson, Pendzik, and Snow also addressed the important topic of research in Drama Therapy in a recent wide-ranging publication, *Assessment in Drama Therapy* (2011). Those who are interested in learning more about drama therapy will find a wealth of information in these timely volumes.

My point of view, then and now, is that, although we all have our biases about what helps people to change and grow, it may not matter so much *what* theoretical orientation one has, as long as one *has* a theory, is well trained with regular and close supervision, and has had one's own therapy. The latter point may turn out to be the most important ingredient that accounts for success in treatment, as recent research, reviewed by Schore (2007), points out.

Schore, a neuroscientist, suggests that those who are right-brained, empathic, and intuitive make better therapists than their left-brained colleagues. This gives further support to those of us who have long urged that all those working in drama therapy (or any field of mental health) have their own individual therapy. It stands to reason that the better we know ourselves, the better we can know and understand others. As we become aware of our own preoccupations and defenses and our blind spots, we are in a better position to make sense of what is going on in us, core issues, and potential transferences to our patients, and we are therefore in a better position to make sense of what is troubling others. Armed with this kind of self-awareness, we can be the kind of empathic, knowledgeable therapist Schore was talking about, able to be of skillful help to others. Thus, the tripartite model that Landy advocated makes sense: training in drama/theatre and therapy, supervised internships, and our own treatment, offering the best hope of being able to help others.

The NADTA organization's Code of Ethics, list of training programs, and requirements to become a Registered Drama Therapist are listed on their website (www.NADTA.org), information that is also listed at the end of this chapter.

EFFECTS OF ATTACHMENT AND A NURTURING ENVIRONMENT ON THE ABILITY TO WORK AND PLAY

What makes it possible for children to be able to engage in dramatic play? And what skills are needed to be a good player? The following examples of two children close in age illustrate the skills of a nurtured child and the play of a child who was damaged by sexual abuse and neglect. Both were born to mothers and fathers who were on drugs during their conception and the ensuing pregnancy. The first child, however, was reared by a loving grandmother after the age of 6 months. The second child was not as lucky, continuing to live with her drug-abused parents.

Case Study A

Three-year-old Arthera carried her baby doll tenderly, talking to it quietly and singing a sweet song. Feeding and burping the baby, she repeated, without awareness, the tenderness and care she received early on, not from her drug-abused and abusing mother, but from her loving "nana" who adopted her at 6 months old. Noticing her therapist watching, Arthera smiled benignly and then turned back to her baby, the two forming a loving unit.

Case Study B

Linda, a 4-year-old child who had been physically and sexually abused, handled her naked baby doll roughly, talking to it in a growling voice. She repeated a pattern of banging the back of the baby's head on the table, while forcefully throwing back her own head and arching her back, laughing hysterically. This pattern was repeated over and over. Putting the toy hypodermic needle into the baby doll's vagina, she laughed even harder, her laughter turning into a scream. Her look at the therapist was defiant, provocative. In a way that was painful to watch, she enacted the unspeakable, unbearable abuse she had received from her grandfather.

The Attachment Process and the Beginning Formation of the Self

From birth, brain development proceeds rapidly, and early experiences contribute to the development of the growth of the mind, stimulated by the mother's attentive care and interaction with the newborn. If all goes well, by 9 months to a year, infants are on their way with a secure base of attachment that is encoded in their implicit memory, which Bowlby (1969) and Stern (1985) called a "working model" of the world and how people interact. The healthy confluence of an attentive mother and a nurturing environment is theorized to be the beginning of a core sense of identity, which culminates in a secure attachment (Cassidy & Shaver, 1999; Schore, 2003, 2007; Siegel, 1999; Stern, 1985, 2004; Winnicott, 1965, 1971).

But as Fonagy and Target (2002) and others remind us, *it is not attachment per se* that is important, but the scaffolding that a secure attachment can provide, making it possible for infants/toddlers to organize their internal state and regulate their sense of emotional well-being. Children who have a healthy sense of self, like Arthera, mentioned earlier, firmly anchored in a secure attachment, are able to develop the skills necessary to be a good player. She can play with her mother, at first; then play alone when mother is nearby; then play with her peers, ultimately engaging in sociodramatic play, using the skills noted later.

But a child like Linda, also described earlier, who has had a life of fear, trauma, and pain, will have great difficulty being able to play, let alone to learn and work. Her traumatic history has prevented her from developing the kind of skills necessary for play: the ability to attend, remember, focus, share, express herself verbally, and especially to contain her inner chaotic world. Linda would need the special help of a drama therapist, counselor, or play therapist to learn to play and self-regulate.

Given healthy development, children would have the following skills, which are needed to be a good player:

1. The ability to *symbolize*—the capacity to "pretend," holding an imaginary visual, motor, and kinesthetic image in mind, while conveying the gist of this inner representation through gesture and emotionally colored speech.

2. The ability to *share with others and delay gratification*, keeping in check anxiety and pressing needs, and having the capacity to find a congenial way to be smoothly integrated into the group or drama, taking an appropriate role.

3. The ability to *convey the emotional essence of the role*, whether it is a scolding mother, crying baby, or an impatient doctor. The capacity to play different roles reflects one's "ego identifications"—the unconscious mental process whereby children temporarily become like another, also taking in the other's feelings. Internalization of these aspects of the outer world, and children's interactions with it, are "taken in" and become the core of the inner self. The ability to take on and play different roles, therefore, is rooted in *identifications and interactions with significant others*.

4. Good-enough *verbal* skills to be understood, whether playing a "good" or "bad" guy, verbally and nonverbally painting a picture of the imaginary other.

5. The ability to regulate feelings and to hold anxiety in check. Erikson (1950, p. 223) commented that as ideas float in and out of consciousness, underlying fears sometimes emerge, out of awareness. If the anxieties are of sufficient intensity, *play disruption* may take place, the play may stop, and children may withdraw.

6. The capacity to have a sufficient *grasp of the boundaries of reality and fantasy*. Gould's concept of *fluctuating uncertainty* (1972) is similar to Erikson's play disruption (i.e., children who are intently involved in play may experience uncertainty about fantasy/reality, what is real/unreal). Unable to keep the "as if" pretend situation in mind, anxious children may stop playing, or act out.

This may seem like a long list of capacities, but keep in mind that early development is complex, with many steps to be negotiated. Children need to learn and practice these skills, which are necessary not only for playing, but for learning and living as well.

Part of the task of drama therapists, and of all who work with children, is to help them to regain the capacity to play. As Winnicott (1965) notes, if children or adults cannot play, then it is the therapist's task to teach them to play, reaching the still-vital part of the self that is accessible through imagination and a personal connection that will make communication possible.

A compelling reason to see the therapist's task as facilitating fantasy and the necessary dramatic play skills can be found in Sara Smilansky's seminal work in Israel. Her research, published in 1968, indicated that many emotionally and/or culturally deprived children need a "play tutor" to help them learn to play, because missing skills will not develop on their own. Additionally, Smilansky's research indicated that being a "poor player" has implications for children's future ability to learn. Smilansky pointed out that the skills gained in dramatic play (as outlined above) are crucial for success in the "school game," where such cognitive and emotional abilities are needed for symbolic thinking, reasoning, planning, and working with others.

DRAMA THERAPY TECHNIQUES

Some, if not most, children engage in improvisational play from the moment of the initial therapeutic encounter. Good players need only an invitation to play, or perhaps the therapist's suggestion that they make up a story from a picture, use a puppet to tell a story, make up a puppet story, or become a character in a fantasy, stimulated by a mask, cape, or soldier's hat. But sometimes children are emotionally blocked, inhibited, or fearful of play. These children need more structured help to begin the therapeutic journey. Whatever the situation, it helps to have interesting materials to catch children's imagination and to begin the play that can lead to a therapeutic alliance.

Having said that, however, it is important to keep in mind that it is *not the materials per se* that are important. Materials are just a means to an end, enlarging the possibility that we can form an alliance with children or adolescents, enabling us to understand and be of help. The goal of drama therapy is to help children feel *psychologically safe enough to express their inner world with its wishes/fears*, giving us a chance to "diagnose" (i.e., understand) and "treat" (i.e., help) them with their painful preoccupations (and defenses against them), perhaps even clarifying the ways they have tried to explain and deal with these problems in the past. What do we need to have—or do—to help children express themselves?

A Play Space and Materials

A playroom, while highly desirable, is often not possible, and many therapists use their offices for play sessions. In such a case, an open bookcase with plastic bins with play materials in an attractively arranged space will let children know, symbolically speaking, "Play is spoken here." It's helpful to remember that although children may begin in one modality (say, through art or clay work), there is often considerable fluidity in the sessions, as images/fantasies in one area often lead to dramatic enactments in another modality. There are no rigid boundaries within *any* of the modalities, and the general rule is that the therapist begins where children are most comfortable, following their lead. The following is a rough guide to the kinds of play materials most children enjoy.

Because young children like water, sand, clay, artwork, dolls, and toys, it is helpful to have some of the following:

- A sandbox (or a large plastic container of fine, washed sand)
- Plastic buckets, spoons, pitchers, and water bottles to be used either with water or wet or dry sand
- Plasticine and clay for modeling, clay-shaping tools
- Art materials with a range of colors and sizes of paper, and markers to use in drawing or painting
- Boy and girl dolls that wet; dolls that can be fed and nurtured (or neglected, abused)
- Miniature life toys, including:
  - Transportation toys: trucks, planes, police cars, fire trucks, ambulances, racing cars
  - Farm animals, fences, stones, wild animals
  - Dishes and pretend food, containers for water for "cooking"
  - Soldiers, war planes, tanks, guns, cowboys, Indians
  - Doctor/nurse kits, fake bandages, play money
  - Miniature family dolls

Children in latency and adolescents enjoy puppets, costumes, and sand/water play as well. The following materials would be useful to have on hand:

- Variety of family and "royalty" puppets, as well as wild and tame animal puppets
- A puppet stage (or a table under which someone can hide to enact a puppet story)
- An assortment of costumes and props (e.g., cloak, robe, soldier's hat, umbrella, cane, sunglasses, scarf, fancy hat)
- Balloons, telephone, aforementioned assortment of art materials, and craft materials to be used for construction projects, such as popsicle sticks, glue, cardboard, and so on

Games in Therapy

In the previous list, there is no mention of games, checkers, or cards, items that are often the mainstay of child therapy. Although I have a few games (i.e., checkers, cards) in my playroom, they are kept in the back of the toy closet, not readily seen by the child. This is because I prefer a more unstructured, open process that is likely to lead into a fantasy enactment, rather than games, which are often used as a *defense* against play. That is, because games with predictable rules often provide a safe, structured refuge from troubling feelings, I prefer not to have them be front and center with other materials. However, the unwritten rule in working with children is that one needs to be flexible and begin where the children are. If the structure of games is needed to help lower children's anxiety, that is where we begin, hoping that as children feel psychologically safer, we can move to more creative materials.

Sometimes, games can be used in a fall-back position when one is in a therapeutic stalemate with patients, and interpretations are either off-base or ignored. In such a situation, one can try to devise a safe, competitive game that will allow children an outlet for possible feared (or projected) aggression, which is sometimes the cause of phobic reactions in treatment. To break an impasse, for example, one could humorously suggest a nonverbal "talking game" with paper and markers: "*You* make a mark, and then *I'll* make a mark. But remember, no talking!" (Rubin, 2005). Or, to try to get through a stalemate, one can also use Winnicott's imaginative "Squiggle" game (1950), or Fraiberg's (1963) "What Pops into your Head?" activity. These are creative attempts to understand and deal with children's unconscious resistance.

Sometimes, puzzled by hurt or angry children who cut off communication, I try to "talk" via a nonverbal form of messaging. Sending a paper airplane flying their way, with a drawing or a verbal message, is an attempt to connect, repair, or try to learn more about what is happening. Usually I get a return plane message, sometimes with an "ugly" picture or an undecipherable message on it. On occasion, however, children have taken pleasure in destroying the airplane, tearing it to little pieces. But, even so, the logjam is broken, aggression is safely expressed, and we are still in touch, albeit nonverbally. Other times, I may try to call children on the telephone. Sometimes they will answer, provocatively, "Police Station! We're coming to arrest you!" Others are happy to have a chance to be passive-aggressive and will answer the phone, only to hang up, banging the receiver! But again, even if this happens, it keeps us "talking" and working on repair of the rupture (Tronick & Gianino, 1983).

DRAMA THERAPY TECHNIQUES WITH DIFFERENT AGES

Preschoolers

Many years ago, Lois Murphy (1956) suggested having a small, portable collection of miniature life toys that could be used in a therapy room, at school, or even in children's homes. Murphy advised the therapist to look at both the *content* of the spontaneous children's play (*what* the play is about), as well as the structure of the children's play (i.e., *how* they play—with clarity or confusion, order or disorder). Murphy believed that the *how* (structure) of the play was more important than the *what* (content), even though the "what" is more compelling and often easier to understand.

Technique

The technique is a fairly straightforward one. The miniature toys are placed in random piles (but grouped in categories together—i.e., transportation toys, animals, etc.) in a circle on the floor. While sitting on the floor, the therapist says: "You can play with these toys in any way you like." With this open invitation, children can begin to explore, while the therapist observes the approach to play, level of autonomy and freedom versus constriction and rigidity, and the content (themes) and form (structure) of the play.

Case Study: Play With Miniature Life Toys in a School

During a school consultation, the principal voiced concern about Elaine, a depressed and anxious kindergartener, asking if I would see her. In a meeting, the parents said that Elaine had been upset since two older cousins came to live with them in their already-too-small house. For several months, Elaine had not been eating or sleeping well, sometimes even sleepwalking. The parents were perplexed.

In the first session, I put the toys in a circle on the floor and invited Elaine, a thin, apprehensive child, to play with them in any way she liked. After inspecting them carefully from a distance, she slowly approached, movements tight and constricted, and picked up the closest toy—a little girl figure and a dog with a chain to "go with" the girl. After a short walk with the dog, Elaine had a larger girl come into the scene, who then pushed the little girl away, and took the dog. Elaine looked aghast, and the play stopped. The symbolic disguise of play, which assures psychological safety, was gone and play disruption was evident.

Seeing that Elaine was immobilized by anxiety, I said to the little girl, maintaining the "as if" of the drama, "Oh my, you wanted to take the dog for a walk, but she took the dog from you?" After a minute or so, making steady eye contact, and with a serious look, Elaine nodded.

In a stage whisper, I suggested that perhaps we could both play, but change roles. She could be the bigger girl; I would be the smaller one. Confused at first, it took a few minutes for her to understand role reversal. But when she, as the bigger girl, came to take the dog, I indignantly said, "Hey! What are you doing? That's not nice!" Startled, Elaine laughed out loud, and then she did it again and again, enjoying the "aggressive" confrontation. Finally, I said to the bigger girl: "Okay, you have a turn, but it's *my* turn first—no pushing me around!" Again Elaine laughed and we replayed the story with a few variations (arguing about a bed, food, a toy), giving this timid child a chance to try on an assertive role.

This brief consultation accomplished two things. First, it verified what was happening at home—that Elaine felt displaced and "unfed/unloved," because the bigger kids (who also felt displaced) monopolized and took away things, maybe especially mom (perhaps symbolically represented by the dog). Clearly something had to be worked out, as mom, the principal, and I discussed. Second, on a theoretical level, one of the core values of play was illustrated in this brief vignette: that Elaine was given an opportunity to turn from passive to active (Waelder, 1933), turning away from the "pushed-around" victim role to a more assertive role, protecting her rights. And, with her mother supporting her in speaking up, the home situation improved.

Sandplay Worlds

Since its conceptualization by Margaret Lowenfeld (1926) (as well as Charlotte Buhler, 1951; Dora Kalff, 1980; and Lois Carey, 1999), sandplay has been widely used in individual and family treatment. Most practitioners follow Buhler's prescribed procedure by using two trays of sand, one wet and one dry, and a multitude of miniature figures, placed on shelves where they can be readily seen. In most "official" miniature sandtray collections, there are people and animal figures, fantasy figures, transportation toys, as well as an assortment of signs, rocks, and shells. The official sandtray assortment is much larger than the smaller miniature toy collection I use, which is closer to that advocated by Lois Murphy (1956) in her Miniature Life Toys Procedure.

It has always seemed to me that the specificity of the sandtray figures may be somewhat constricting, whereas fewer toys leave more to the child's imagination. Additionally, I use only one sandbox, not two (a wet one and a dry one), as Buhler prescribed. If children want to add water to their "world" constructions (or even "flood" the sandbox), they can do so; the water dries out fairly quickly and has the added benefit of giving us the opportunity to explore the symbolic meaning of the flooding. Once children make a world, they are asked to tell a story about it, as in the following example.

Tommy's Story

Tommy, a 7-year-old African American boy, was almost nonverbal as he entered the playroom. A smart but underperforming child, he was referred because he seemed sad, played alone, and was seemingly uninterested in learning, an attitude that was quite different from that of his 9-year-old sister. On a few occasions, however, he exploded at school, lashing out at others, sometimes hitting them. His perplexed, overwhelmed single mother said with annoyance, "I don't know *what* to do with him—always got a chip on his shoulder—like it's *my* fault his father left or something! And every once in a while he blows up, terrible blowups, and then he won't talk for days. And sometimes, too, he poops in his pants. I don't know what it is."

In the playroom, Tommy seemed indifferent to the many materials, but he eyed the sandbox warily. Told he could play if he wished, he turned his back to me and nonverbally fingered and smoothed the soft sand, enjoying the tactile feel. Saying that kids could use either wet or dry sand, I pointed to the squirt bottles, saying he could use those if he wanted water.

Before long, Tommy made a mountain in the sandbox, with a mother figure close to the top and a little girl (called "sister") midway down. Far at the end of the sandbox was a village with little houses, fences, and some rocks. Completely absorbed, Tommy spoke little and only stopped momentarily to get more water to shape the mountain. When he finished, I said it was as though he made a "world" picture and asked him, "Could you tell a story about it?" Without hesitancy, he said, "Well, the mountain's gonna explode and kill all the people in the village down there . . . with hot stuff." Asked what might then happen to the mom and the sister, he said, "Umm, they'll probably get killed first by the hot stuff, too, 'cause they're so busy fightin', they didn't see the mountain was gonna blow up." Then he shrugged and said, "Oh, well" (as though to suggest that it wasn't his fault).

Although Tommy continued in weekly therapy for six months, this first session provided psychological clues about what might be troubling him. Mom and sister did indeed fight a lot, as Tommy said. In later sessions when the play was repeated, it became clear that Tommy missed his dad and "blamed" his mom and sister for their fights (and perhaps blamed himself, too, for his own blow-ups and "poopy" accidents). In subsequent sessions, Tommy continued to elaborate the theme of family aggression, ultimately saying, "Sometimes I get so mad I wanna punch somebody!" Finding an appropriate outlet for his own aggression helped him better control and moderate his own feelings, enabling him, in several family sessions, to tell his mother how much he hated the fighting and how much he missed his dad ("Too many girls around! Not enough guys."). Once again we are reminded of Erikson's comment about a child finding a "trusted adult" to whom he could show the "secret hate," to find play peace.

Puppet Play

Sometimes preschoolers engage in puppet play, but generally this activity is more appropriate for children in latency, preadolescents, and even adolescents (Irwin, 1983, 1991; Irwin & Shapiro, 1975). Although puppets can initially be costly, a variety of puppets can be purchased over time, and they are quite durable, lasting for many years, unlike supplies that get used up. Because children like to pretend that the story is "pure" make-believe, it helps to have something to serve as a stage for the children to hide behind (i.e., a table, cardboard box, or a play structure).

It is important to have a *range* of puppets in *different categories* (Irwin, 1983, 1991; Irwin & Shapiro, 1975; Portner, 1981). This can include family puppets (mother, father, children); royalty puppets (king, queen, prince, princess); symbolic "bad" parent figures (witch, ogre, skeleton, pirate); animal puppets (domestic and wild, including a friendly dog as well as a scary dragon); and occupation puppets (doctor, police officer). Because puppets portray "forbidden" wishes, kids love to use fierce, scary puppets (i.e., witch, bad guy) as well as contrasting friendly puppets, of both people and animal types. In general, it is better not to have character puppets (Snow White, Evil Stepmother) in order to help children "make up a story you've never seen or heard before . . . one you've made up all by yourself."

Procedure

The puppets are spilled onto the floor while the therapist notes which are selected and which rejected, because the selection process is important. Once the child has picked out four or five puppets for the story, he or she goes under the table or behind the stage, and the therapist announces, "Ladies and gentlemen, welcome to the land of make-believe. We're about to have a special television puppet special by Master John (or Miss Jane—either a real or made-up name), so sit back and get ready to see the show!" (Gardner, 1985).

Then as part of the audience but also as the announcer, the therapist warms up the child by asking a few brief questions about the story elements: *who* (characters in the story), *where* (the setting), and *what* (the plot). After the child has introduced the characters one by one, the therapist engages in a brief dialogue with the main puppets, helping the child feel comfortable with the make-believe that is about to follow: "Good day, your Majesty. Is this your kingdom?" "Oh! A pirate! Gosh, what do you *do*, Mr. Pirate?" "Mr. Skeleton? Oh my, is this the land of the dead?"

Interviewing the Puppets After the Story

Once the story begins, the therapist sits back and takes rough notes of the action. After the story is over, the therapist maintains the make-believe by interviewing the puppets (not the child!), asking sensitive, but general questions about the plot, action, characters, and possible motives in the story. In the last part of the inquiry, one can ask more direct questions to determine if the child has some psychological clues about how the puppet story may be linked to his or her own life: "If you could, is there anyone you would really *like* to be in the story? Anyone you *wouldn't* like to be?" (And perhaps one might ask why or why not.) Then, to determine the story's theme, the therapist can ask, "If the people in TV land were to learn something from this story, what might it be?" And "If you could give your story a name, what might you call it?" One can also ask the child if he or she has any ideas where the story came from, which is really an invitation to explore the deeper meanings of the puppet story. There is a great deal to be learned from this procedure, including the child's preoccupations and defenses against them, as well as the possibility of gaining a glimpse into cognitive and emotional capacities (Irwin, 1983, 1991; Irwin & Shapiro, 1975). A video of a family puppet interview by Elaine Portner, PhD, a family and drama therapist, is available through www.expressivemedia.org

Varied Themes, Reflecting Past and Present Anxieties

By giving children a variety of puppets from which to select the characters for their stories, one taps into current as well as past worries. Sometimes the stories are very realistic, like Tommy's, portraying fighting parents. This led him to talk about the impending divorce in the family.

Sometimes the stories reflect ongoing troubling wishes, fears, and unresolved issues, like when George played a story about pirates who robbed and tried to steal the King's gold. Of all the many stories that could be told, one wonders why George selected *this* particular theme of aggression and robbery. In subsequent sessions, George spoke more openly about revolt in the kingdom and the wish to kill the "mean king." All of this was grist for the mill.

Sometimes the puppet stories tap into bad dreams, as when Brian chose a skeleton and dragon that terrorized all of the animals in the forest. When I wondered how he happened to think about such a scary story, Brian first talked about a *Frankenstein* movie, and then said, "I've been thinkin' about it ever since. Sometimes I can't even go to sleep!" Eventually Brian said he thought Frankenstein was a little like his father, who was "mean and scary. Sometimes I think he might even hurt us, maybe kill us, but . . . I know he *won't!*"

These stories provide an opportunity for children to project forbidden wishes and fears onto the "safe" puppets. But more importantly, they allow children to verbalize their suppressed/repressed thoughts, because one can *safely* talk about the "King's" bossiness, or fear of the Frankenstein-like father, or even a child's wish to kill the fierce dragon. But one cannot talk openly about such wishes connected to people in the family whom children also love and needs However, just because the wishes are out in the open does not mean that the psychological work is done. What's left is the crux of therapy, helping children to figure out what the story has to do with their life and what they can do to make things better for themselves.

Costumes: Another Way Children Can Safely Project Hidden Wishes

It often helps to have a box of costume pieces as well as some props. After a session or two, when children feel more comfortable, they can be invited to look in the prop box and find something that interests them and make up a story. Patty loved the toy cash register that rang a bell when she struck the numbers. This led her to suggest that we play "toy store." I was to be a mean mother, she said, who bought lots of toys for my younger girl, but only "messy, dirty" toys for my older child, who interestingly, was said to be 10, the same age as Patty. This story eventually developed into Patty's taking on the role of the mean mother herself in dramatic play. She tormented me, the mother-customer, and then she put me in prison, poisoned me, and threatened me with fierce animals that would eat me up. This kind of play is like "the royal road to the unconscious," as Bettelheim said. It doesn't matter that the story changed; that suddenly the "good" shopkeeper turned into the "bad tormenter" shopkeeper/mother; or that I am suddenly the "bad girl" who deserves to be punished by the cruel mother. Unraveling the play meanings is the crux of therapy, as Patty was slowly able to see that she was enraged with her once-good mother, turned "bad" when she adopted and fussed over the new kid in the family, ignoring Patty, the once-good older kid. But again, while the discharge of rage was illuminating and certainly provided relief, what is still to be worked out are the ways that Patty can come to terms with, and learn to manage and accept, the new family constellation.

Similarly, 9-year-old Janine, whose drug-addicted mother had mostly abandoned her, was captivated by a pair of high heels. Putting them on, she "became" her mother, dancing and drinking, locking me—her child—out of the house, later yelling, "Get your smelly butt to bed!" Taking the assigned role of the daughter, I pleaded with "mom" to let me in the house, saying I was scared and didn't know what I had done wrong. Because Janine had a more fragile ego, with fewer satisfying years behind her, helping her to develop self-regulation and achieve emotional distance was much harder than it was for Patty. Nevertheless, the pure unadulterated joy and catharsis of the play helped her to make significant but slow changes in her life with her aunt, a more tolerant and loving caretaker than her immature mother, who had indeed once locked Janine out of the house in the midst of a drug-fueled party, to be rescued by the neighbors.

In short, one needs only a few props and perhaps some pieces of material to suggest characterization. A fancy piece of cloth served as a robe for 14-year-old Jimmy, who became a dictatorial king, sentencing me, his child, to death. My crime? Poor school grades—not surprisingly, also a heated topic of contention in Jimmy's house. Whatever feelings and ideas are inside of the child, waiting to be expressed, may be *denied, displaced*, and *symbolically projected* into the play, often distorted and magnified. These defense mechanisms are often the heart of the work in drama therapy (and in play therapy), helping to explain why this modality is psychically safe and successful. In this sense, drama therapy treats children's whole brain: the right hemisphere, full of potentially powerful, confusing feelings, and the left hemisphere, which can help them find words and ideas to make sense of the play.

If one begins with a telephone, bell, purse, gun, soldier's hat, whatever, a story soon gets formed around the symbolic projections and distortions that are nonetheless derivatives of children's unconscious fantasies. After that, it is up to the therapist to help structure the play, keep it pretend but psychologically safe, and "give form to the feeling" (Langer, 1953). And, if asked to take a role in the drama, it is very important that the therapist maintain therapeutic distance and be careful not to unduly contaminate the play. This might mean liberal use of the stage whisper, such as when asking for direction: "What happens next?" or, "What does she say?" This helps to assure that the child is in the lead, and it stays in the child's control as *his* fantasy, and not the therapist's!

CONCLUSION

This chapter briefly traced the roots of drama therapy, linking this expressive modality to psychoanalytically oriented play therapy and child analysis, as well as other forms of action-oriented treatment (psychodrama, Gestalt, theatre games, etc.), all of which emphasize spontaneity and understanding. In drama therapy, the drama is the easy part—the therapy is the harder part. The latter refers to the task of helping children with the task of *making meaning*: that is, making sense of the play and connecting it to their life. And that is why the therapist needs to have an equal balance of training and understanding in both drama and therapy.

SPECIALIZED TRAINING AND RESOURCES

Becoming a Registered Drama Therapist (RDT)

The purpose of these Standards of Registration is to identify as Registered Drama Therapists those people who have: expertise in dramatic, theatrical, and performance media; understanding of psychotherapeutic processes with different populations in a variety of settings; experience with the integration of the artistic and psychological aspects of drama therapy; and professional work experience in the field of drama therapy, mental health, and special education.

Registration Requirements

To qualify as a Registered Drama Therapist (RDT), the applicant must:

1. Meet all of the educational requirements
2. Meet all of the basic eligibility requirements
3. Meet all of the requirements for additional training/work experience

Education Requirements

The applicant must have *either* a:

1. Master's degree or Doctoral degree in Drama Therapy from an NADTA-accredited college or university

OR

2. Master's degree or Doctoral degree in a field related to Drama Therapy (i.e., drama/theatre, psychology, counseling, special education, social work, occupational therapy, recreation therapy, art therapy, music therapy, dance/movement therapy, etc.) from an accredited college or university and completion of the Alternative Training Education requirements under the supervision of an RDT or Board Certified Trainer (BCT)

In addition, the applicant must have completed:

- Drama Therapy Internship consisting of a minimum of 300 direct-client contact hours with a minimum of 30 hours of supervision by a Registered Drama Therapist, credentialed creative arts therapist, credentialed special educator, or credentialed mental health professional and an additional 470 hours of additional internship hours (including, but not limited to, staff meetings, preparing for sessions, contact notes, reviewing professional materials, and other administrative work).
- A maximum of 50% (150 hours) of the direct-client contact time may be one-on-one contact, while the remaining 50% (150 hours) must be group work.
- During the internship, applicant must have worked with a minimum of two different populations (e.g., emotionally disturbed, physically disabled, adolescent, elderly). It may be that the applicant is able to work with two populations at one internship site. If not, the applicant may need to do an internship at two different sites. The total hours of internship does not change in any case (i.e., 800 for one or for both counted together).

Basic Eligibility Requirements

The following are eligibility requirements to become an RDT:

- *500 hours of drama/theatre experience.* This may include acting, directing, and/or improvisational work studied or performed in a college, community, or professional setting.
- *1,000 hours of paid experience as a drama therapist.* You must be supervised by a Registered Drama Therapist, credentialed creative

arts therapist, or credentialed mental health professional or special educator.

- ○ Not more than 40 hours per week can be counted.
- ○ The 1,000 hours may begin to be accrued before students graduate from their MA program in Drama Therapy once all of their coursework and internship hours are completed (and while they are working on their thesis). This is the same for alternative training students working on their MA in a related field. Alternative training students who had already completed a Master's or Doctoral degree before entering alternative training may begin to accrue hours once their core drama therapy coursework and their internship is completed.
- ○ *However,* whenever the hours begin to be accrued, the rule for one calendar year from when the MA degree was granted stands for the application process.
- ○ If you have acquired drama therapy experience in a position that was unpaid, it can be counted toward the paid work hours; however, you must have a letter from a representative of the agency to document that the position was recognized by the agency as professional and which provides a brief narrative justification for the nonpaid status.

- • You cannot apply for the RDT until at least a calendar year after your MA degree is granted (however, if your degree was granted in May of the previous year, you may apply for your RDT in the March 15th cycle as the RDT will not become official until May).
- • You must be a member of NADTA for at least one year prior to applying for registration along with proof of membership.
- • You will need to write a one-page essay describing your work and your philosophy of drama therapy in relation to the NADTA definition of drama therapy.

Additional Work/Training Experience

Five hundred hours of additional training/work experience is also required. This may include:

- Additional hours of drama therapy internship over and above the 800 required hours.
- Additional hours of work experience over and above the 1,000 required hours.
- Additional hours of clinical training in drama therapy or a related therapeutic field. This can include workshops, conferences, postgraduate institutes, practica, institutes, or apprenticeship programs.
- Up to 100 hours of personal psychotherapy within the last five years. To document this you will need a signed letter from your therapist noting that you attended the stated hours of psychotherapy and the dates it occurred. No additional personal information is to be included in the letter.

Some applicants may want to utilize college- or university-level coursework done in addition to their MA degree. In accordance with the National Post Secondary Education Standards, a one-credit course is worth 45 hours of clock time, a two-credit course is worth 90 hours of clock time, and a three-credit course is worth 135 hours of clock time.

Postgraduate and Alternative Training Programs

These universities and training centers offer courses in drama therapy that can be taken to fulfill the requirements of alternative training or as supplementary postgraduate training in specific methods and approaches to Drama Therapy.

Alternative training students are not limited to the schools on this list but may find courses at other institutions and may take training courses at several different schools. Students who do not live near a training program may be able to complete their training by taking courses locally, online, and through intensives. The Board Certified Trainer (BCT) is a member of the faculty of the National Association for Drama Therapy, and to ensure they receive credit toward the RDT (Registered Drama Therapist) requirements, current and potential alternative training students are encouraged to establish a relationship with a BCT, who will advise the student about course requirements and eligible coursework. Students are also encouraged to read the alternative training manual to evaluate whether the course content and instructor's credentials meet the alternative training requirements.

Antioch University (Seattle, WA)
MA in Psychology with Concentration in Drama Therapy
Contact: Bobbi Kidder, MA, RDT/BCT
http://www.antiochseattle.edu/academics/psychology/dramatherapy-
    overview.html

The Center for Living Arts (Oakland, CA)
Director: Armand Volkas, MFT, RDT/BCT
www.livingartscenter.org

Creative Alternatives of New York (New York, NY)
Program Director: Heidi Landis RDT/BCT, LCAT, CP, CGP
Director of Training: Lucy McLellan RDT/BCT, LCAT
www.cany.org

Drama Therapy Institute of Los Angeles (Los Angeles, CA)
Director: Pam Dunne, PhD, RDT/BCT
www.dramatherapyinstitutela.com

Institute for Developmental Transformations (New York, NY/San
    Francisco, CA)
Training Director (NYC): Navah Steiner, MA, RDT, LCAT
Training Director (CA): Randy McCommons, MA, MFT, RDT/BCT
www.developmentaltransformations.com

Kansas State University (Manhattan, KS)
MA in Theatre with Concentration in Drama Therapy

Director: Sally Bailey, MSW, MFA, RDT/BCT
http://cstd.k-state.edu/Theatre/Pages/Graduate/DramaTherapy.html

Lesley University (Cambridge, MA)
MA in Expressive Therapies
Instructor and Coordinator of Psychodrama/Drama Therapy Specialization: John Bergman, MT, RDT/BCT
http://www.lesley.edu/academics/programs/expressive_therapies.html

Rehearsals for Growth (RfG) (Leverett, MA)
Director: Daniel J. Weiner, PhD, RDT/BCT
www.rehearsalsforgrowth.com

Nova Southeastern University (Ft. Lauderdale, FL)
MS in Interdisciplinary Arts/Drama Therapy
Track Director: Norman J. Fedder, PhD, RDT/BCT
www.schoolofed.nova.edu/iap/dramatherapy_program.htm

Omega Transpersonal Drama Therapy (Boston, MA)
Director: Saphira Linden, MA, RDT/BCT, LCAT, CP
www.omegatheatre.org

Soul Studies Institute (Stuart, FL)
Director: Wendyne Limber, RDT/BCT
www.soulstudies.com

Presence Center for Applied Theatre Arts (Charlottesville, VA)
Director: Mecca Burns, RDT/BCT
www.presencenter.org

Accredited Schools

California Institute of Integral Studies (CIIS)
1453 Mission Street
San Francisco, CA 94103 USA
Phone: (415) 575-6230
Renee Emunah, PhD, RDT/BCT
Program Director and Professor, Drama Therapy Program
Accredited by the North American Drama Therapy Association
   since 1991

Concordia University
Master's Programme in Creative Arts Therapies
1455 de Maisonneuve Blvd. West
Montreal, Quebec H3G 1M8 CANADA
Phone: (514) 848-2424 ext. 4790
Stephen Snow, PhD, RDT/BCT
Associate Professor and Coordinator, Drama Therapy Option
Department of Creative Arts Therapies
Accredited by the North American Drama Therapy Association
   since 2000

New York University
Program in Drama Therapy
35 West 4th Street, Suite 777
New York, NY 10012-1172
Phone: (212) 998-5258
Robert Landy, PhD, RDT/BCT
Professor and Director
Drama Therapy Program Department of Music and Performing Arts
   Professions
Accredited by the National Association for Drama Therapy
   Association since 1989

REFERENCES

Bettelheim, B. (1987, March). The importance of play. *The Atlantic Monthly*, 35–46.

Bornstein, B. (1949). *The Analysis of a Phobic Child*. Psychoanlytic Study of the Child, Vol. 3/4, 181–226.

Bowlby, J. (1969). *Attachment and loss: Vol. 1. Attachment*. New York, NY: Basic Books.

Buhler, C. (1951). The world test: A projective technique. *Journal of Child Psychiatry, 2*, 4–23.

Carey, L. (1999). *Sandplay therapy with children and families*. Northvale, NJ: Jason Aronson.

Cassidy, J., & Shaver, P. R. (1999). *Handbook of attachment: Theory, research, and clinical applications*. New York, NY: Guilford Press.

Durning, C. (2012, December 28). Obituary. *New York Times*.

Erikson, E. (1950). *Childhood and society*. New York, NY: W. W. Norton.

Fonagy, P., & Target, M. (2002). Early intervention and the development of self-regulation. *Psychoanalytic Inquiry, 22*, 307–335.

Fraiberg, S. (1963). Technical aspects of the analysis of a child with a severe behavior disorder. *Journal of American Psychoanalytic Association, 10*, 338–367.

Freud, S. (1955/1909). Analysis of a phobia in a five-year-old boy. In J. Stachey (Ed.), *The standard edition of the complete works of Sigmund Freud* (Vol. 10). London, England: Hogarth.

Freud, S. (1955/1920). Beyond the pleasure principle. In J. Strachey (Ed.), *The standard edition of the complete works of Sigmund Freud* (Vol. 18). London, England: Hogarth.

Gardner, R. (1985). *Therapeutic communication with children: The mutual storytelling technique*. Northvale, NJ: Jason Aronson.

Gould, J. (1972). *Child studies in fantasy*. New York, NY: Quadrangle Books.

Grotowski, J. (1965). *Towards a poor theatre*. New York, NY: Simon & Schuster.

Hug-Hullmuth, H. von (1921). On the technique of child analysis. *International Journal of Child Analysis, 2*, 287–305.

Irwin, E. (1983). The diagnostic and pretend use of play. In C. E. Schaefer & K. J. O'Conner (Eds.), *Handbook of play therapy* (pp. 148–173). New York, NY: Wiley.

Irwin, E. (1991). The use of a puppet interview to understand children. In C. E. Schaefer, K. Gitlin, & A. Sandgrund (Eds.), *Play diagnosis and assessment* (pp. 617–635). New York, NY: Wiley.

Irwin, E., & McWilliams, B. J. (1974). Play therapy for children with cleft palate. *Children Today, 3,* 18–22.

Irwin, E., & Shapiro, M. (1975). Puppetry as a diagnostic and therapeutic technique. In I. Jakab (Ed.), *Transcultural aspects of psychiatric art* (pp. 86–94, Vol. 4). Basel, Switzerland: Karger.

Johnson, D. R., & Emunah, R. (2009). *Approaches to drama therapy.* Springfield, IL: Charles C. Thomas.

Johnson, D. R., Pendzik, S., & Snow, S. (2011). *Assessment in drama therapy.* Springfield, IL: Charles C. Thomas.

Kalff, D. (1980). *Sandplay* (2nd ed.). Santa Monica, CA: Sigo Press.

Klein, M. (1932). *The psychoanalysis of children.* London, England: Hogarth.

Landy, R. (1982). Training the drama therapist: A four-part model. *The Arts in Psychotherapy, 9,* 91–99.

Langer, S. (1953). *Feeling and form: A theory of art.* New York, NY: Scribner.

Lowenfeld, M. (1926). *Play in childhood.* New York, NY: Wiley.

McDougall, J., & Lobovici, S. (1969). *Dialogue with Sammy: A psychoanalytic contribution to the understanding of child psychosis.* New York, NY: International Universities Press.

Moreno, J. (1946/1959/1962). *Psychodrama* (3 Vols.). Beacon, NY: Beacon House.

Murphy, L. (1956). *Methods for the study of personality in young children* (Vol. 1). New York, NY: Basic Books.

Perls, F. S. (1969). *Gestalt therapy verbatim.* Moab, UT: Real People Press.

Piaget, J. (1962). *Play, dreams and imitation in childhood.* New York, NY: W. W. Norton.

Portner, E. (1981). *You can learn a lot from a lobster!* Video of a family puppet session. Accessed at: www.expressivemedia.org

Rubin, J. (2005). *Child art therapy: 25th anniversary edition.* Hoboken, NJ: Wiley.

Schore, A. N. (2003). *Affect dysregulation and repair of the self.* New York, NY: W. W. Norton.

Schore, A. N. (2007). Developmental affective neuroscience and clinical practice. *Psychoanalytic Research,* 6–15.

Siegel, D. J. (1999). *The developing mind: Toward a neurobiology of interpersonal experiences.* New York, NY: Guilford Press.

Smilansky, S. (1968). *The effects of sociodramatic play on disadvantaged preschool children.* New York, NY: Wiley.

Spolin, V. (1975). *Improvisation for the theatre: Theatre game file.* St. Louis, MO: Cemrel.

Stanislavski, C. (1936). *An actor prepares*. New York, NY: Theatre Arts Books.

Stern, D. N. (1985). *The interpersonal world of the infant: A view from psychoanalysis and developmental psychology*. New York, NY: Basic Books.

Stern, D. N. (2004). *The present moment in psychotherapy and everyday life*. New York, NY: W. W. Norton.

Tronick, E. Z., & Gianino, A. (1983). Interactive mismatch and repair: Challenges to the coping infant. *Zero to Three: Bulletin of the National Center Clinical Infant Program, 5*, 1–6.

Waelder, R. (1933). The psychoanalytic theory of play. *Psychoanalytic Quarterly, 2*, 208–224.

Winnicott, D. W. (1950). *Through pediatrics to psycho-analysis*. London, England: Hogarth Press.

Winnicott, D. W. (1965). *The maturational processes and the facilitating environment: Studies in the theory of emotional development*. New York, NY: International Universities Press.

Winnicott, D. W. (1971). *Therapeutic consultations in child psychiatry*. New York, NY: Basic Books.

Integrating Play Therapy and Sandplay Therapy

RIE ROGERS MITCHELL, HARRIET S. FRIEDMAN, AND ERIC J. GREEN

INTRODUCTION

Both play therapy and sandplay therapy provide children with the opportunity to use symbols (i.e., toys and other materials) to communicate their thoughts, feelings, fantasies, and experiences nonverbally to an accepting and supportive therapist. For most children, play is the only way to express and communicate their difficulties; often, words are not used in therapy to express inner issues until adolescence.

Sandplay therapy, based on the psychological principles of C. G. Jung (1956), was developed by Swiss therapist Dora Kalff, who studied at the Jung Institute in Zurich and with Margaret Lowenfeld in England. Sandplay therapy is sometimes referred to as a "creative arts therapy," as well as a play therapy technique. Certified sandplay therapists mostly use sandplay with adults (Friedman & Mitchell, 1992), though it can be used with children.

When children enter the *free and protected space* (Kalff, 2003) of a playroom that contains a variety of small and large toys, sand, and other play equipment, their imagination is immediately stimulated, and the natural healing powers of the psyche are enlivened, allowing them to express and "play through" the issues that have brought them to treatment. "Free" because children can create whatever they desire in the sand, and "protected" because the therapist is present to protect the children and the space from intrusions, harm, and other distracting events. The presence of the therapist, who understands the literal and symbolic meaning of the toys, supports positive development and growth of children through either silently witnessing the creation of a sand picture or actively playing with children during play therapy.

THERAPEUTIC PLAY

Although most children are naturally drawn to the toys in a playroom, many child therapists have found that an introduction to the playroom and toys facilitates and sets the tone for therapeutic play. Some therapists, for example, introduce the playroom by saying (with an "awe-inspired" voice), while motioning to the room and toys, "This is a very special place where you can play and do almost anything you like here." Some add, "I will tell you if you can't do something." Thus, children know that there are some limits in the room. Typical limits are developmentally appropriate rules, such as not hurting self or others, inappropriate destruction of property, and so on. The therapist may then suggest that children look or walk around the room to choose what would be fun to do.

When introducing sandplay, directions are somewhat more specific than in introducing play therapy. Sandplay therapists often say, "Here are two trays filled with sand. As you can see, one tray is wet; the other tray is dry. Would you like to feel the sand?" Then, "Here (gesturing to shelves of miniatures) are miniature toys and other objects you can use in the sandtrays. If you like, you can use these objects to make a picture in the sand." Later, if children create a sand picture, sandplay therapists often add, "After you leave today, I am going to take a picture of what you've made in the sand, if that is all right with you, so you can later see all of your sandplay pictures." Usually children are uninterested in seeing pictures of their old sandplay trays; they are busy creating new aspects of their lives. However, some child clients return as adults to review their sandplay pictures.

Some therapists prefer a more organic introduction to sandplay therapy. They wait to see how children intuitively use the sand, water, and miniatures. If a child is playing with only the sand *or* the miniatures, the therapist may mention that the miniatures and sand can be used together to create a picture in the sand.

Sandplay therapy, within the context of play therapy, allows children to create an imaginative world by placing miniatures in a tray (19.5 inches by 28.5 inches with a depth of 3 inches), half-filled with fine-grained, sterilized white sand and painted blue on the inside to give the impression of water and/or sky. Dora Kalff (1971), the founder of sandplay therapy, said that sand represents instinct, nature, and the healing power of Mother Earth. The miniatures on nearby shelves are a stimulus to children's imagination and represent many aspects in their world. The children's choice of miniatures helps the therapist to symbolically understand the issues that are displayed in the sand.

Normally, two trays are available in sandplay therapy, so children will have a choice of wet (damp) sand or dry sand. A container of water is often placed nearby, so more water can be added to the sand. The therapist usually sits a little behind the client and takes notes on the order of the miniatures placed in the tray and their movement, client comments, and therapist's thoughts. Some therapists draw a picture of the sand pictures for their notes. Photographs of the sandplay scene, taken by the therapist after children have left the therapy session, provide a permanent and ongoing record of children's internal processes. Thus, sandplay serves as a window into the children's inner world, and provides the opportunity to express a myriad of feelings, unspoken thoughts, and even the unknown. Sandplay scenes may be created quickly, in as little as 10 minutes, or take the entire therapeutic hour. Usually, a sandplay picture is not created at every therapy session; it is the child's choice when, and if, to use sandplay.

After giving the child an opportunity to examine the toys and miniatures during the first session, some therapists ask, "Would you like to make a picture in the sand now?" The reason for inviting the child to create a sand picture during the first or second therapy session is that playing in the sand often helps the child feel more comfortable in the new play therapy environment. In addition, the content of the tray and the process the child uses in creating a sand picture can provide useful information about the child. For example, Kalff (personal communication, July 1978) said that a first tray may suggest: (a) how the child feels about therapy, (b) the child's relationship to the unconscious, (c) the nature of the problem, (d) the solution to the problem, and (e) in our experience, the first tray can also give information about the child's relationship to the therapist. Also, because children under 8 years old tend to create trays similar to other children of the same age, it is possible to acquire a deeper understanding of the child's developmental level from the child's first sandplay creation, especially if the tray deviates from the norm (Bowyer, 1970).

SANDPLAY IN A PLAY THERAPY SETTING

Sandplay is one of many expressive arts therapy interventions that a therapist can use within the play therapy environment. Both sandplay and play therapy are considered to be mostly nonverbal and nondirective creative techniques. However, children do seem to talk more during play therapy than sandplay therapy, probably because in play therapy the children and therapist have face-to-face interaction and often play together; relating and reacting to each other is an important part of play therapy. In contrast, children using sandplay have the opportunity to connect to their own internal self without verbal involvement of the therapist. In sandplay the focus is strictly on the relationship to oneself, so that the sand pictures reflect what is happening within children's inner world. Thus, children usually create sand pictures mostly in silence with the therapist sitting nearby, observing the play.

Although both play therapy and sandplay therapy can serve as a window into children's internal world, sandplay adds structure to the relatively unstructured play therapy environment. For example, in sandplay, children are asked to create a picture within the confines of the sandtray using miniature toys that are usually not used in play therapy. In child-centered play therapy, the therapist typically does not suggest the nature or outcome of the play; children play freely with any item in the playroom, as long as they stay within the traditional limits of play therapy. However, some children, especially young children under 8 years old, prefer to play freely in the sand and not make a picture.

After a play therapist actively engages with children in play therapy, they may decide to create a sandplay picture. At this point, the therapist normally changes his or her role from an active participant in the play to a silent observer of the sandplay process. This allows children's own natural imagination to be the guide in creating sandplay pictures.

It is important for the therapist to realize that the developmental level of the child affects how she or he uses sand and miniatures. Bowyer's 1956 research (summarized in Bowyer, 1970) on the influence of age on the scenes created in a sandtray indicates that young children (2 to 3 years old) usually demonstrate little or no focus; their trays are chaotic and disorganized, and they typically use only a small portion of the tray. Sand is often dropped and thrown outside of the tray.

Bowyer in 1956 (Bowyer, 1970) also found that children 4 and 5 years old often use only a small portion of the tray; however, they sometimes move toys around the tray, while fighting, making noises, and speaking for the miniatures. The sand is mostly used for burying and unburying miniatures. A fixed picture in the sand is unusual for children at this age.

At ages 6 and 7, according to Bowyer in 1956 (Bowyer, 1970), children normally begin to use the full space of the tray and expand their ability to control the way they create the tray, with transport (e.g., cars, trains) often being used. Children 8 and 9 years old use sand in a constructive way, creating roads, waterways, and buildings. Most of the tray is used, and miniatures are arranged to represent action rather than having to move the miniatures around the tray. At 10 and 11 years old, children frequently show control in the tray by using fencing. The peak age for use of fences and signs in the tray is 10 years old. By 12 years old, sand pictures are often indistinguishable from those created by adults (Bowyer, 1970).

When a play session is over and the child leaves the playroom, the therapist (with the child's previous permission) photographs the child's work in the sand. A photographic record of the child's sandplay pictures provides permanent and ongoing information about the child's therapeutic process.

Role of the Therapist

The therapist's role in sandplay is to establish a *free and protected space* in which children can relax and allow their internal state to be accessed and expressed. This experience is similar in feeling to Winnicott's (1965) description as that of *being alone in the presence of the mother*, who is present and accepting, but not intrusive.

Play therapists often participate in the child's play if they are invited by supporting, mirroring, and sometimes modeling and encouraging play behavior (Green, 2012). In contrast, play therapists who are also sandplay therapists generally sit near the child, but to one side, as the tray is being created, often taking notes, but not being involved directly in the child's play in the sand. This close proximity can help establish trust and rapport beyond just verbal interaction, including an unconscious connection between client and therapist. When a safe space is provided by an empathetic therapist, children can truly relax, access their imagination, and allow the internal world to be safely experienced and expressed in the tray.

It is important that the therapist knows how to tolerate in silence the uncertainty of not always consciously knowing what children are communicating. Watching and listening without using words may be unfamiliar and difficult for some therapists; however, silence is important in sandplay. "Silent listening," while maintaining an attitude of openness and acceptance, helps create a safe and protected space that leads to children's spontaneous, new internal directions.

Through the process of playing in the sand and creating pictures using miniatures and/or actively playing outside of the sandtray, children can experience psychological and cognitive changes. Play allows children to express themselves nonverbally, retrieve memories of early childhood experiences, as well as become calmer and more at peace. To illustrate this therapeutic process with children, David's work in play therapy and sandplay therapy is discussed in the following section.

Case Study

David began therapy when he was 7 years, 6 months old and in the second grade. During nearly four years of almost weekly therapy sessions, he created a series of 25 sandplay scenes and participated in many play therapy activities. Some of these activities are discussed, along with six of his sandplay trays. During his time in therapy, David moved from an anxious, frightened child to a more relaxed and confident preteen.

My first impression of David was of a skinny, frail-looking wisp of a boy. He seemed so anxious, helpless, and depressed that my first impulse, which I (Mitchell) had to control, was to reach out and take care of this weak and lethargic child. Although David was normally silent at home, in his first session he talked openly about his experiences and feelings, and from the beginning he was committed to regularly attending therapy sessions.

Initially I did not know that his fears and fantasies had entrapped his life energy; thus, his energy was unavailable to him to use in his outer life of school and relationships. Early on, he told me in many ways that he felt different from others.

Background Information

Before David started therapy, I met with his mother; his father was unable to attend this session. She reported that David's symptoms included stomach cramps, which appeared during school months but disappeared during vacation. He had also had sleep problems since birth, including insomnia, sleep terrors, and sleepwalking. When he was stressed, he had strong emotional reactions, including rage, tears, and once, when he was 6 years old, a threat of suicide. Additional symptoms concerned his mother: thumb-sucking at home but not at school; excluding himself from social contact with his peers (even when his peers actually wanted to be with him); unfocused speech patterns; and underachievement at school, including not finishing his work and daydreaming. His mother commented, "The impression is that David is slow, but actually he is bright. I have a bright boy who doesn't know how to communicate it to the world."

David is a middle child with two sisters. His older sister, an intellectually gifted teenager, was actively involved with friends and extracurricular interests. His younger sister was born about 18 months after David. His mother thought that perhaps David was not given as much attention as he needed, since their births were so close together. However, she said that she feels a very special connection to David, and she is much more protective of him than she is of her daughters.

David's father is a police officer. His mother described her husband as having a "horrible temper." She said, "He gets angry unexpectedly, especially at David. My husband is not physically abusive, but when he gets angry and yells, it's as though he hates us. Most of the time, he worships the children."

The extreme worry that David's mother carried began even before his birth, when the results of an ultrasound test suggested that David was missing one leg. At his birth, he was immediately taken away from her without reassuring comments from the doctor. While waiting to see her newborn son, her fears magnified and grew to incredible heights. Later, when David was finally brought to her, the doctor said, with apparent relief, "He's fine, just fine." However, the doctor's words and David's normal appearance did not relieve the terror she felt, and she continued to carry that feeling with her in interactions with David.

Another important dynamic in understanding David's issues is that he had a very porous and intuitive nature, which left him with few defenses against the highly charged issues in the home and in his inner and outer worlds. For example, David was described by his mother as "very perceptive." According to her, if David said something was going to happen, it would happen or had already happened. She cited this example: One evening his police officer father was on a stake-out, waiting for suspects in a burglary to appear so he could arrest them. At home, without any knowledge of what his father was doing, David suddenly became very upset and told his mother, "Dad is chasing some criminals, and they pointed a gun at him." Later, when she told her husband what David had said, he verified that David's description of the arrest was correct. His mother told me that this type of knowledge was typical for David, and he intuited happenings in other situations as well, not just with his father.

I came to realize that David's withdrawn and inhibited behavior was supported by a whole spectrum of difficulties: his mother's anxiety and fear for David, which resulted in her becoming overprotective; his father's anger and rejection of David because of his timidity, which made David feel even more frightened, worthless, and helpless. David's own sensitive nature both caused, and was a result of, his intuitive and close connection to his mother and his father's angry and negative behavior toward him.

Therapeutic Process

During our first therapy session together, David best expressed his view of the family dynamics when he drew a picture of his family doing something a kinetic "Draw a Family" [DAF]. It showed his sisters and parents riding in a motor boat, looking straight ahead, while the boat pulled David along behind on waterskis. No one was paying attention to him. David did feel very much alone, although his being alone was largely his own choice.

One of David's favorite activities in play therapy was to "play fight," with each of us holding a *bataka* (i.e., a heavily padded paper cylinder with a handle at the end). In addition to "fighting," David enjoyed trying to knock my *bataka* out of my hands, while I tightly grasped it lengthwise between my hands. When he was able to hit it hard enough, so it flew out of my hands, he would laugh with glee and pump his muscles. He also enjoyed playing board games, especially when he won, and he loved playing with puppets; they could express what he could not.

Later in therapy, we explored the stream and small hills outside of my office. We even played a little soccer and baseball, although he soon found out that I was no challenge. Mainly, toward the end of therapy, we talked about his life, the challenges he experienced with his father, the demands of his schoolwork, and his growing enthusiasm and abilities in athletics. Throughout his therapy he often created sandplay pictures, which not only chronicled his growth and development but also allowed him to express what was happening consciously and unconsciously in his life.

During his therapeutic process, David created 25 sandplay scenes. Six of David's sandplay scenes are discussed as follows. For each sandplay picture, the following information is given: David's name for the sandplay and his age. These were created from the age of 7.5 to just past 12 years old. The sandplay scenes represent various aspects of his development during his nearly five years in therapy. David named all of his sandplay scenes, which is unusual for children his age.

In the center of the sandtray, David placed a bandaged man on a stretcher, with two doctors, a male and a female, standing on each side of the stretcher. David moved the sand so that these miniatures appear

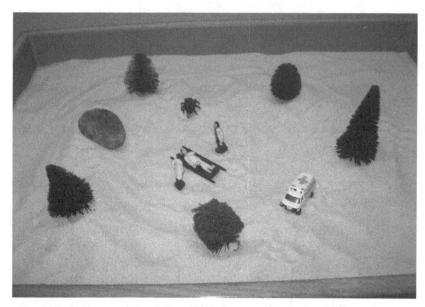

Figure 5.1   MASH Unit (7.5 Years Old)

contained within a womblike space. Nearby and to the right is an ambulance. Above the stretcher and slightly to the left are three objects that
form a triangle: a spider, a rock, and an autumn tree. Four green trees
surround the medical scene.

David's situation is depicted clearly in this tray, suggesting a strong
(and perhaps porous) connection to the unconscious. The tray has a
somewhat barren and empty quality; its starkness suggests isolation,
desolation, and suffering, which is what David was experiencing at both
home and school. Trays that have an empty quality, depict injury, and
contain prone figure(s) suggest the possibility of early wounding.

The prone, bandaged man on the stretcher is similar to David,
wounded and helpless, both caught between his parents and yet needing their assistance. Help is available in the form of two doctors (male
and female) and the ambulance. I noted that David placed the doctors
and ambulance near to where I was sitting, and David was standing as he
created his tray. The visible sign of the ambulance helping the distressed
figure on the cot was a potentially positive sign, as it may have been
depicting David's psyche showing it had the capacity for self-care or
inherently knew when distress was abounding and healing was needed.

With all of the other barren landscape and shadowy figures in this picture, this one symbol gave rise to hope that David did have some inner resources to rely on to help him in his trajectory to self-healing.

The spider, located above the wounded man, suggests potential for further wounding. The spider is most often viewed symbolically as a poisonous mother symbol. In David's outer life, he was caught in his mother's overanxious web of worry about his well-being. I believe her constant uneasiness and overprotective behavior was experienced by David as being caught and held back. David may have felt caught in the web of anxiety from his mother's projections and overprotectedness, similar to a fly being unsuspectingly tangled in freshly spun spider web.

As I viewed the tray, additional questions came to mind: What do the four trees in the scene symbolize? Natural energy and growth? Or perhaps they represent the four other people in his family? Does the ambulance and doctors, placed near to us, indicate a positive transference and that perhaps help is now available?

The dying evergreen tree at the back of the tray concerned me, as did the rock and the spider, which seemed to be threatening the wounded man. I wondered about David's potential to resist change and growth

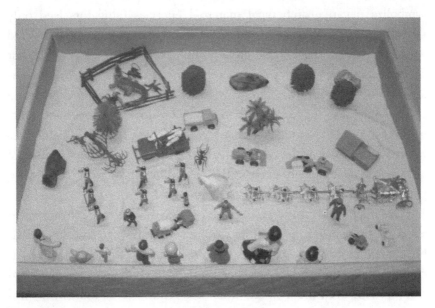

Figure 5.2   The Big Parade (7.6 years old)

in therapy. I hoped that the four green and vibrant trees represented David's life force and would help him connect to the energy he needed to move forward. This may have depicted, early on, a glimpse of his *self-healing archetype* (the ability of a child's psyche to generate symbols and for the child to follow them toward healing).

In this tray, help is again available. The same wounded man (from the first tray) is now in a jeep (left/middle) with the doctor and nurse. Presumably, he is being taken to a hospital for treatment. The parade (representing David's psychological movement) includes a horse-pulled gold coach, which is being protected by the police and soldiers from intrusion by the bicycle riders and the black spider (behind the doctors in the jeep).

Work machines (a cement mixer, dump truck, and tractor) suggest that internal work is going on. I was pleased to see that David placed a white shell (near the front of the tray in the middle) in the midst of the parade. The shell is one of the eight emblems of good luck in Chinese Buddhism, signifying a prosperous journey.

With the penned alligator and spider (top/left), I could see that David was now in the process of containing elements that may have hindered his development in the past. The alligator and spider are considered to symbolize negative archetypal maternal energies (alligators feed only the babies that snap at flies; spiders eat their young). The snow-covered wintergreen trees suggest that growth and development are possible, but the trees are currently dormant; thus, change may not happen immediately. The rock from his initial tray (top/right corner) and the driftwood (middle/left) also suggest that change may be slow (i.e., rocks and driftwood take time to form and change). However, the four small palm trees nestled together near the top/middle of the tray suggest the possibility of growth and development even in the most difficult of circumstances, for palm trees are strong and highly resilient.

I was happy with this tray, because I always hope to see movement in a second tray, suggesting that the psyche is beginning to shift and possibly change in a positive way. Also, the movement was ordered and non-chaotic, suggesting the ego was beginning to potentially constellate and regroup. However, the rock and driftwood reminded me that, while progressive elements (the parade and trees) are alive and active in David's

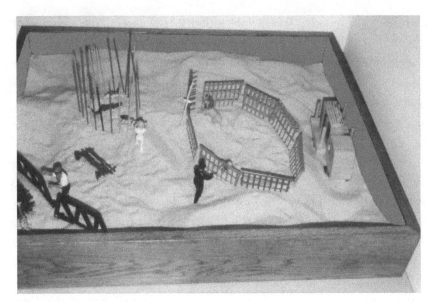

Figure 5.3   Testing the Animals (age 9.0)

process, regressive and resistant aspects are also evident in this tray; the rock suggests resistance and inflexibility. Now that I look back on this tray, I see that the natural piece of driftwood symbolized David's therapeutic process (i.e., that transformation would occur but through a natural process that would take some time).

At 9 years old, David was doing somewhat better in school, and he was a member of a Little League baseball team. He created a tray he named "Testing the Animals." In this tray, David placed two males and a female (he called them "scientists") in front of enclosures that housed untamed animals. David said that the scientists were studying the animals' behavior.

The scientists in the sandtray suggest that it is now possible for David to have the ability to think about and develop a more objective attitude about his situation. The primitive and younger aspects of his psyche— the alligators, giraffe, lions, and bear (in the cage on wheels, located on the right side of the tray)—are now separated. This is a necessary separation if David is to disentangle himself from his enmeshed family.

It may be possible for the lion to escape from its cage through the break in the fence. If this "break" were to happen for David, it would then be possible that David's wild, primitive energies could either over-whelm him or bring him the considerable primitive strength he needs.

A giraffe, on the left-front side of the tray, is eating, taking in nour-ishment. As the tallest species, a giraffe has a wide range of vision and symbolizes objectivity of thought. Objectivity is necessary in David's life, helping him rise above his family situation of both overprotection and rejection.

Also, the appearance of mandalas, or circular formations representing the formation of the Self, appeared in this sand picture. This is typically indicative of a child's psyche entering the Alchemical phase, *nigredo* (or "charring of the soul"), where boundaries are built to protect and bolster the defenses of the fragile ego in preparation for the next phase of the psychological "hero's journey." When mandalas appear spontaneously in children's symbols, in Jungian terms, it represents the ego-Self axis (the child's psychological and often tenuous connection between the inner [affect] or "Self" and outer [behavior] or "Ego"), seeking balance before it begins the next part of the heroic journey.

Almost immediately after David made this sandtray, his behavior and sandtrays moved in a new direction. Now, with clearer vision and an objective ego, David takes a more differentiated stance. He seemed

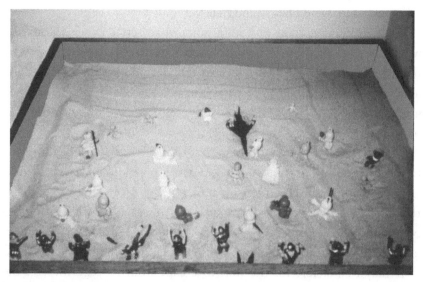

Figure 5.4   Babies Take Over (age 10.1)

better able to use his fine mind, which aided him in his task of separa-tion and individuation and freed him to embark on his necessary hero's journey, as well as to integrate his stronger, more positive capacities in his everyday life.

One year later, David made the tray he named "Babies Take Over." After smoothing the sand, he randomly placed the babies, with two of them sitting on a jet plane. He positioned rifles beside some of the babies. Next, David lined soldiers along the front of the tray with their hands up in the air, facing the babies as if they were surrendering.

As David drew barely visible lines in the sand, linking the men to the babies, he told me that the lines were electric wires, which the babies could pull and electrocute the men if they moved. He said, "The babies are tired of being bossed around. They have become bad now. Their pictures are on the Most Wanted posters, so the guys have come after them."

I was pleased to see that David (symbolized by the babies) was dis-playing so much new energy. However, many questions came to my mind as I reflected on the tray, and I wondered what had been awak-ened in David. Perhaps, he had discovered new independence and strength? If so, would this new power endanger his new energy (i.e., the babies)? I also gave some consideration to the possibility that this was a regressive tray. However, I was more convinced that David was finally gathering his strength to deal with the destructive masculine energy in his home. This was evidenced by his drawing clear demarcations in the tray, or archetypal "lines in the sand," representing, in Jungian terms, an activation of the psychic energy emanating from the *animus* (male) archetype.

Around this time, at 10 years old, David was willing to discuss his relationship with his father in more detail than ever before. He told me about his father's unpredictable temper and how scared he felt when he was younger. Now, he found he could relate to his father through sports. They both enjoyed watching sporting events together on television. He seemed to be gathering strength despite his mother's overprotectiveness. However, the babies in the tray suggested that this energy was still very new, quite young, and undeveloped. I knew that he would continue to need support in his development.

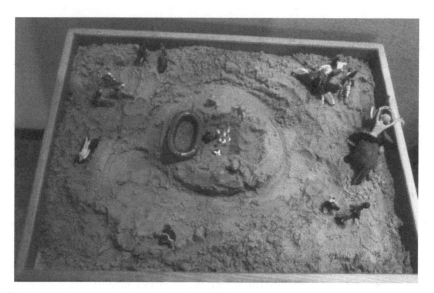

Figure 5.5   Fight for the Crown (Age 12.0)

In play therapy, David was spreading his wings, and we often ventured outside of the office, taking walks, fording small streams, and climbing nearby hills. He shared with me his success in baseball; he was chosen the league's Most Valuable Player. Around this time, he was also performing at a high academic level. His school identified him as "gifted," and he entered that program.

For many months, David did not create sandplay scenes. Then, one day, he walked into the playroom and immediately went right to work in the sand and made two trays.

As David was making the tray, he told me the following story: "These babies are in trouble. The Indians (upper/left and upper/right) are trying to steal their crown and candles" (the six white candles are in the candelabra in the center of the tray, along with the crown). "But, the babies have a plan—if the bad guys get closer, the babies will take the candles and crown and put them into the lifeboat. Then the babies will use their special powers and lift the lifeboat into the sky away from the bad guys."

The central organizing principle, the Self, is symbolized by the circular area that David carefully delineates in the middle of the tray. With this emergence, David is now able to display a stronger sense of self. Within this area, he places the crown, candelabra, silver lifeboat, and four babies. Four is the number of wholeness. The lifeboat is a symbol of help, rescue, and safety. The candelabra, near the lifeboat, offers warmth, energy, light, and consciousness to the situation. The crown is a visible sign of success and of *crowning* achievement. This circular shape, or mandala, illuminated the numinous transformation occurring within David's inscape.

Despite the threatening and possibly destructive forces of the unconscious nearby (i.e., the Indians), David is now able to separate and protect himself from their potential invasion. That is, the tortured figure on the elephant is leaving the tray, and the wounded man takes a more distant position. He is aided by the four clever and imaginative babies, who represent newly emerging aspects of himself.

After completing the previous sandplay, David began to play with the sand in the other tray. I asked if he wanted to create another picture. He responded with a "yes." As he quickly made this tray, he explained that the two baseball teams have traveled through time and represent the best teams from their worlds.

In the symbol of the baseball diamond, it was clear to me that David's internal Self had at last become consolidated and connected to his ego (his outer life); now both his inner and outer worlds are more

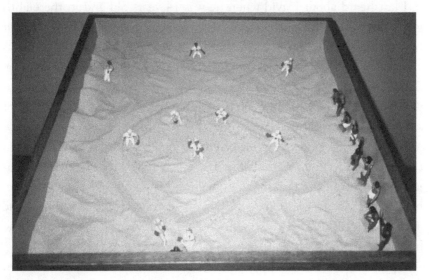

Figure 5.6   The Baseball Game (Age 12.0)

connected. I watched with pleasure as David quickly and with confidence placed a baseball team on a diamond he outlined in the sand. The diamond shape is a powerful symbol of the totality of the Self. Through the game of baseball, on a diamond-shaped field, David has found an age-appropriate connection to the outer world. The opposing team of cavemen, waiting on the sidelines, symbolizes the archaic, primitive, and archetypal aspects of David that were symbolically being "sidelined" as more complex dispositions and healthier ego-defenses were constellating. In the past, these aspects have attempted to take over to detract and pull him in a regressive direction, often successfully. I was pleased to see that the cavemen were now on the sidelines.

CONCLUSION

After David's 17th sandplay, he continued in therapy for quite a while, using the time to paint, play games, and talk together. He created eight more sandtrays, which suggested further consolidation and strengthening of his independence and ego. With his newfound awareness, David then worked in conjoint therapy with one of his sisters to deal with their family concerns. He was performing very well in school when he terminated therapy.

I last heard about David when he was 14 years old and in the eighth grade. He was successfully involved in baseball and football. That year he won the league's Most Valuable Player award in football, and he was chosen for the USA youth baseball team scheduled to go to Beijing, China, that summer. He was liked and respected by his teachers and was popular with his peers, although he still enjoyed being alone and did not socialize easily with others.

David's mother now described him as a quiet person, who is calm and consistent under the pressure of sports. She believed that he was particularly astute in understanding and meeting his own needs. For example, he decided not to participate in basketball that year (even though he also excelled in that sport), because he needed leisure time between the busy football and baseball seasons.

It appears that David, as a teenager, was able to access his own inner strength, while his outer life was a natural reflection of his own distinctive abilities and interests. As he further matures, there will be more room for his excellent intellectual abilities to emerge. Whatever his future, I am certain that David will live it in his own unique way.

SPECIALIZED TRAINING AND RESOURCES

Selected Books on Sandplay

> *Sandplay: Past, Present and Future* by Harriet S. Friedman and Rie Rogers Mitchell (Routledge)
>
> *Supervision of Sandplay Therapy* by Harriet S. Friedman and Rie Rogers Mitchell (Routledge)
>
> *Sandplay: A Psychotherapeutic Approach to the Psyche* by Dora M. Kalff (Temenos Press)
>
> *Sandplay: Silent Workshop of the Psyche* by Kay Bradway and Barbara McCoard (Routledge)
>
> *Sandplay and Storytelling: The Impact of Imaginative Thinking on Children's Learning and Development* by Barbara A. Turner and Kristin Unnsteinsdottir (Temenos Press)

Selected Books on Integrating Play Therapy and Sandplay With Children

> *Inscapes of the Child's World* by John Allan (Continuum)
>
> *Handbook of Jungian Play Therapy* by Eric J. Green (Johns Hopkins University Press)
>
> *Sandplay: Therapy With Children and Families* by Lois J. Carey (Jason Aronson)
>
> *Sandplay Therapy in Vulnerable Communities: A Jungian Approach* by Eva Zoja (Routledge)

Selected Sandplay Therapy DVDs

> *Sandplay: What It Is and How It Works* by Gita Morena (Sandplay Video Productions)
>
> *Jungian Play Therapy and Sandplay With Children* by Eric J. Green (Alexander Street Press)

Helpful Links

The Sandplay Therapists of America
www.sandplay.org/links.htm

International Society for Sandplay Therapy
www.isst-society.com

Canada: www.sandplay.ca
Germany: www.sandspiel.de
Israel: www.sandplay.co.il
Italy: www.aispt.it
Netherlands: www.sandplaynederland.org
Switzerland: www.sgsst.ch
United Kingdom: www.sandplay.org.uk

Colorado Sandplay Therapy Association: Research & Training
    Institute
www.sandplaytherapy.org

Center for Jungian Studies of South Florida
www.jungcentersouthflorida.org

The Israeli Sandplay Therapist Association
www.sandplay.co.il

Certification as a Sandplay Practitioner

The following information is taken directly from the *Handbook of Certified, Teaching and Practitioner Member Requirements and Procedures for Sandplay Therapists of America,* which can be accessed at www.sandplay.org/pdf/STA_Handbook.pdf

Prerequisites and Training Requirements

The SANDPLAY PRACTITIONER category of membership responds to an expressed need of STA members to recognize professionals who have completed a personal process and some sandplay training. This membership category is offered to those interested in offering sandplay within the scope of their license and training. It is also recognition of partial fulfillment of the requirements to become a Certified Sandplay Therapist (CST) and/or Certified Sandplay Therapist–Teacher (CST-T). A Sandplay Practitioner may provide sandplay in his or her work without supervision and advertise appropriately (e.g., on business cards) that she or he is recognized by Sandplay Therapists of America as a Sandplay Practitioner. A personal sandplay process or training hours provided by a Sandplay Practitioner cannot be counted toward membership in STA at the practitioner or certified levels of membership.

Prerequisites
Applicants must:

- Hold, in the United States, a valid state license or credential as a mental health professional or a professional license, credential, certificate, or equivalent in an allied field, such as nursing, teaching, or spiritual direction.
- Hold a commitment to in-depth inner development and insight as gained through analysis and/or psychotherapy.

Training Requirements
- Complete a sandplay process with a STA/ISST Certified Sandplay Therapist (CST) or Certified Sandplay Therapist–Teacher (CST-T). An honest, transformative personal sandplay process is the most significant, foundational requirement of the training sequence. The process must occur with a CST or CST-T after that individual has achieved certified status.
- Complete a minimum of 36 hours of education in sandplay with a CST-T or at an STA-sponsored conference, seminar, or workshop, including 18 hours of an introductory course in sandplay.

Twelve (12) of the 36 hours may be earned through field-tested, STA-approved online courses.

- Participate in group consultation with a CST-T for a minimum of 25 sessions in which the applicant presents at least five hours of sandplay case material or in individual sandplay consultation for a minimum of 15 hours or in a combination of group and individual consultation sessions for a total of 20 sessions. If an individual applicant selects a combination of individual and group consultation sessions, at least two hours of every 10 hours of group consultation must be presentation hours by the applicant.
- Applicants are required to seek consultation from someone other than the therapist with whom they completed their sandplay process.
- Work with a minimum of three clients or students per week, who engage with sandplay on a regular basis, for a minimum of one year (nine months for school counselors) under the consultation of a CST-T.
- Applicants may select an STA certified member as advisor during their training process (please see Applicant/Advisor agreement under Certified Requirements and submit Form 6).

Certification Requirements of the International Society for Sandplay Therapy

- A personal process in Sandplay Therapy with an ISST member that precedes, if possible, a regular course of training.
- Theoretical training of a minimum of 100 hours of participation in training seminars in the tradition of Dora Kalff that is based on the principles of the psychology of C. G. Jung.
- Two written seminar papers, at least 10 pages in length, but not more than 20 pages, with 1.5 line spacing. At least one paper must include clinical sandplay material.
- Supervision of practical work in individual and group sessions, with at least two different supervisors. The total number of supervision hours is determined by each National Society (e.g., Sandplay Therapists of America), with a minimum of 80 hours of individual and group supervision with a Teaching Member.

Of these a minimum of 30 hours must be individual supervision. Fifty (50) hours of group supervision will be acceptable provided the student presents his/her own material on at least 10 occasions within the group supervision hours. In the view of ISST, the supervisor should be different from the personal process therapist.

- One completed case study of at least 30 to a maximum of 50 pages of text with 1.5 line spacing. The case study must be read and evaluated by three ISST Teaching Members, one of whom should be of a National Society different to that of the applicant. The applicant's personal sandplay therapist and the supervisor on the case cannot be one of the readers. The reader will provide an evaluation report of the case study to the advisor and to the candidate. The case reader's fee is determined by the National Society.

Select Sandplay Trainings in the United States

Sandplay Therapists of America Annual Conference: www.sandplay .org/training_conferences.htm#Conferences

Dee Preston-Dillon: http://sandplayvoices.blogspot.com

Rosalind L. Heiko: http://www.drheiko.com/training/sandplay-training -heiko

REFERENCES

Bowyer, L. R. (1970). *The Lowenfeld world technique*. Oxford, UK: Pergamon Press.

Friedman, H. S., & Mitchell, R. R. (1992). Future of sandplay: Responses from the sandplay community. *Journal of Sandplay Therapy*, 2(1), 77–90.

Green, E. J. (2012). The Narcissus myth, resplendent reflections, and self-healing: A contemporary Jungian perspective on counseling high-functioning autistic children. In L. Gallo-Lopez & L. Rubin (Eds.), *Play-based interventions for children and adolescents with autism spectrum disorders* (pp. 177–192). London, England: Routledge.

Jung, C. G. (1956). Symbols of transformation. In *Collected Works*, Vol. 5, p. 31. London, England: Routledge.

Kalff, D. M. (1971). *Sandplay: Mirror of a child's psyche*. San Francisco, CA: Browser Press.

Kalff, D. (2003). *Sandplay: A psychotherapeutic approach to the psyche*. Cloverdale, CA: Temenos Press.

Winnicott, D. W. (1965). *The family and individual development*. London, England: Tavistock.

6

Working With Children Using Dance/Movement Therapy

Mariah Meyer LeFeber

INTRODUCTION

Movement is a language. We all learned to relate on a nonverbal level before starting to communicate verbally. Thus, this nonverbal language of the body is especially powerful for children, who communicate, navigate relationships, and interact with their environment through movement. An early, healthy connection with their bodies enables children to develop a strong sense of self and dynamic sense of both their body image and physical boundaries. For all of these reasons, dance/movement therapy is a highly effective modality for working with children.

This chapter introduces the field of dance/movement therapy, specifically as it relates to working with children. An overview of the field is covered, as well as general goals for working with children and case studies that exemplify these goals. Children are a unique population for the work of a dance/movement therapist, because the limited verbal abilities of children may make it more difficult for them to reach out and express themselves. When words fail, dance/movement therapy fosters children's ability to relate, communicate, and connect on a nonverbal level. Dance/movement therapy utilizes body movement as both a method for assessment and a treatment modality.

DANCE/MOVEMENT THERAPY: PROCESS AND PROCEDURES

As defined by the American Dance Therapy Association (ADTA), dance/movement therapy is "the psychotherapeutic use of movement as a process which furthers the emotional, social, cognitive, and physical integration of the individual" (American Dance Therapy Association, 2008). Dance/movement therapy emerged as a discipline during the 1940s and is an effective treatment for people with developmental, medical, social, physical, and psychological impairments (Levy, 2005). This expressive form of therapy is a bridge linking creative expression and psychological theory (Kestenberg, Loman, Lewis, & Sossin, 1999).

When working with children, dance/movement therapy allows for an environment that is simultaneously structured and freeing. A loose structure provides the boundaries needed for children to feel safe, while the nature of the work—meeting children where they are and building each session in the present moment—allows for as much freedom as a client desires. Dance/movement therapy provides the space for children to explore and discover their bodies while unlocking their potential for creativity. Children are encouraged to find themselves in a supportive environment where there is no "right" way to express or create (Canner, 1968). This creates an affirming environment, where children feel "heard" on a kinesthetic level and are able to experience the value of belonging. Ultimately, dance/movement therapy provides both a bridge for contact and a medium for reciprocal communication (ADTA, 2008).

Research and Effectiveness

A growing body of research supports the power of the modality of dance/movement therapy as an effective vehicle for change and growth. Much of the research done in the field can be found in the *American Journal of Dance Therapy*. At the 2007 annual conference for dance/movement therapists, an international panel considered the crucial nature of early intervention for diagnosis and the prevention of future pathology by offering a panel of therapists working with children using dance/movement therapy. The panel included dance/movement therapists working with children in Israel, Spain, Canada, Germany, Japan, Korea,

Greece, Argentina, France, Finland, Egypt, Sierra Leone, India, and Haiti. Across the many countries and cultures, panelists reported that their research indicated common strengths for the use of dance/movement therapy regardless of location, including, "strengthening communication across cultures; bridging language differences; aiding in trauma recovery and treatment of severe mental disturbances and disabilities; rebuilding generational and societal systems; emphasizing and teaching good parenting" (Capello, 2008, p. 35).

A research study conducted by Enid Wolf-Schein, Gene Fisch, and Ira Cohen (1985) studied the use of nonverbal systems in children with autism and other developmental delays. The study concluded that "dance/movement therapy should be considered an intervention for persons with both autism and mental retardation since there are indications that deviations in nonverbal behaviors do contribute to the overall pathology of the individuals" (Wolf-Schein et al., 1985, p. 78).

More recently, Lily Thom utilized dance/movement therapy within a preschool curriculum in order to address socioemotional development. Thom asserted that through dance/movement therapy, the young students made connections between their bodily feelings and conscious appraisal of their emotions. Through the movement and emotion study inherent in the practice of dance/movement therapy, "the children developed the language, movement and collaboration skills to create an expressive representation of their ideas and impulses" (Thom, 2010, p. 110). This integration, in turn, fostered their personal senses of self and equipped them to deal with social, physical, and cognitive challenges.

Currently in the field of health and psychology, neuroscientists have been increasingly interested in the presence and impact of mirror neurons on mental health and relationships. Regarding this research, Cynthia Berrol notes, "a keystone of the therapeutic process of dance/movement therapy, the concept of mirroring is now the subject of neuroscience. The domains of mirror neurons currently under investigation span motoric, psychosocial and cognitive functions, including specific psychological issues" (Berrol, 2006, p. 303). Dance/movement therapy inherently engages this mirror neuron system in the brain, for both those moving and those witnessing the movement of others. Therefore, dance/movement therapy has the unique potential to unlock and develop some deficient areas in an individual's mirror neuron system through the process of movement.

Theoretical Framework

A few basic principles form the guiding theory of dance/movement therapy. These overarching tenets of the field include the beliefs that (a) behavior is communicative; (b) personality is reflected through movement; (c) changes in movement eventually lead to changes in personality; and (d) the larger an individual's movement repertoire, the more options individuals have when it comes time for them to cope with the environment (Kestenberg et al., 1999; Meekums, 2002). When embodying these tenets while working with children, many find it helpful to work within the structure of Chacian-style dance/movement therapy.

Marian Chace was a pioneer in the development of the field and built a framework and theory for dance/movement therapists based on four major classifications:

- *Body action* focuses on the actual physical movement of the body and the utilization of this movement to increase an individual's body awareness (i.e., sense of where their body is in relation to space, or an awareness of the physical sensations they are experiencing in different parts of the body).
- *Symbolism* includes the ability of an individual to conceptualize, release, and build acceptance through the use of imagery, fantasy, recollection, and enactment.
- The *therapeutic movement relationship* is key to the work of a dance/movement therapist. The therapeutic movement relationship utilizes the movement between therapist and client to build communication and foster trust. A consistent, supportive, and accepting atmosphere is used to begin the process of relationship formation, along with the following: mirroring (reflecting rhythms, patterns, and vocalizations expressed by the client), empathic reflection (reflecting, or attuning to, the physical movement qualities and intensity expressed by an individual), eye contact, touch, vocalizations, props, and rhythmic body action (ADTA, 2008; Erfer, 1995). In particular, props can be helpful

when working with children because they are concrete and tangible, thus serving as a connecting medium between client and therapist.

- *Rhythmic group activity* is the process of utilizing rhythm to modify extreme behaviors, help regulate emotion, facilitate group cohesion, and support expression of thoughts and feelings in a controlled manner within a group (Chaiklin & Schmais, 1993; Levy, 2005).

In addition to these four classifications, Chace created a general group or session structure. The structure is broad and fluid, allowing therapists to adapt it according to the specific needs of each client. It is powerful because it provides a holding space for clients that is comforting yet loose enough to lend itself to the creativity of the moment (i.e., as opposed to being overly programmatic or stifling). This structure includes three parts: body warm-up, theme exploration and development, group closure and processing. Each of these sections allows clients to experience and process in different ways, contributing to a cohesive session as a whole.

During the body warm-up, the initial contact is made between therapist and client(s), and the emphasis is on body action, physically mobilizing individuals, and inviting them to build an awareness of what is happening in their bodies. Observing this process allows the dance/movement therapist to assess a client's present situation and needs, and also gives clues for what might need to be worked on during the theme exploration and development portion of the session. The actual practice of dance/movement therapy relies on the observation of movement behavior as it emerges in relationship, and this begins to unfold for the dance/movement therapist in the body warm-up section (Adler, 2003).

Chace believed that theme development is when the deep learning and processing occurs, as a therapist guides a client into symbolic movement and expands on themes presented in the body warm-up (Chaiklin & Schmais, 1993). Dance/movement therapists are trained to understand, reflect, and eventually expand on the nonverbal expression of their clients. This ability to take tangible movement experiences and guide them into deeper symbolic expression is a cornerstone of the field.

The group closure and processing section is imperative to a cohesive dance/movement therapy session. This time allows for a verbal reflection on the experiences within the session (for those clients who are able), a review of any skills acquired during the session, and some sort of closure or ending to the session. This time allows for temporary closure to the experiences of the session, which can be grounding for clients and secure a sense of safety (Chaiklin & Schmais, 1993).

When working with children, the use of Marian Chace's four classifications and the stability of the consistent group structure provide clients with a sense of comfort that allows their creativity and self-expression to thrive (Loman, 1995). By meeting them at this primary, nonverbal level, the dance/movement therapist is able to help expand and foster communication skills. The resulting improved ability to communicate, on both verbal and nonverbal levels, in turn increases children's self-awareness and ability to cope both with their environment and within relationships.

Goals

When considering the subject of dance/movement therapists working with children, there is an endless array of possibilities. Dance/movement therapists work with children in group and individual settings, in general and special education, in public and private schools, and in mental health settings. Dance/movement therapists' approach may be as diverse as the populations they work with and may include expressive movement, storytelling and role-playing, creative dance, and other movement experiences, both structured and improvised (ADTA, 2008). Because of the vastness of possibilities, my focus in this section is geared toward my personal experience in working with children with developmental delays. The goals and following case studies are suggested with this specific population in mind.

Before working on any specific goals, and akin to Chace's emphasis on the therapeutic movement relationship, the initial and overarching goal for dance/movement therapists is to reach out and meet a child at his or her functioning level. Once this relationship has been established, it serves as a consistent guiding principle behind the work and emerges in the balance between the physical and relational. In the dance/

movement therapy setting, relationships occur as a byproduct of the body in action, and physical movement flourishes because of the trust built within the therapeutic relationship. When the physical and relational aspects of the work are in balance, movement truly can serve as a language for universal communication.

With this relationship in mind, we consider some specific goals and examples. Although each individual child presents with unique needs and challenges, a handful of goals are generally applicable. The first goal is to *increase sensorimotor and perceptual motor development*, directly targeting the motor deficits often faced by children with developmental delays (ADTA, 2008; Erfer, 1995). By working from a standpoint that is both expressive and functional, dance/movement therapists can use simple vocabulary and movement to stimulate perceptual, gross, and fine motor skills. An example of this is teaching children the perceptual concept of "in and out" by having them physically move inside of a space (e.g., a hula hoop) and then outside of that same space. Through the gross motor movement (which can be expressive and of their own choosing), the children experientially learn the concept, which can then be generalized to other areas.

The second goal for dance/movement therapists working with this population is to help clients *improve their socialization and communication skills*. As the therapeutic relationship discussed earlier grows, clients increase their ability to interact as part of a group and communicate (verbally or nonverbally) within that group. Steps toward meeting these goals include increasing eye contact, participating in shared rhythmic activities with engagement (and independently whenever possible), recognizing and responding to group members, increasing proximity to the group, decreasing a need for interpersonal distance, developing trust, and forming an understanding of self as opposed to the others outside of the self (ADTA, 2008).

Although these social and communication goals can be met through several modalities, dance/movement therapy is unique because the steps toward these goals can all be experienced on a kinesthetic level. For example, in group rhythmic activity, group members move together with similar rhythms, intensities, and physical tensions. This extension of movement throughout the body helps clients to integrate what may be a fragmented sense of self (Levy, 2005). Building small movements into total body activity helps build cohesiveness and a sense of grounding not only for people as individuals, but also for their identity as group members. The similar rhythmic and movement patterns allow all clients to feel that they belong on a nonverbal level. This sense of belonging can be especially powerful for children who struggle to communicate on a regular basis. Although they may find it difficult to communicate their experiences verbally, when they create a rhythm in their bodies (e.g., stomping, clapping, or drumming) that is then followed and matched by the therapist and/or group members, they experience a sense of being heard and accepted on the nonverbal level.

Thirdly, building off of the growing understanding of self versus others, dance/movement therapy works to *foster body awareness and nurture a client's individual self-concept*. By reflecting a child's movement nonverbally and then translating what is seen into simple language, the dance/movement therapist positively verbalizes how the child appears, inherently improving his or her body awareness or body image. For example, when warming up, a therapist might say to a child, "Oh, I see you moving your shoulders up and down," which allows the child to begin connecting the felt experience of the movement with the verbal, conscious awareness of what is occurring in time and space. The simple verbalizations, or the noticing of what is going on, also help structure the experience for the participant (Loman, 1995). As an added benefit, this verbalization of action naturally increases the movement repertoire of clients (applicable to goal one), as they are exposed to not only the conscious experience of their own movement but also that of the others in the room.

Body awareness and a positive body image are imperative, as the two combined form a foundation for a basic understanding of the self. Not only does the development of body awareness parallel sensorimotor development, but the movement experience also helps children to orient to their space, their own bodies, and the others in the room. This orientation occurs on both an internal (self-to-self) and external (self-and-others) level. Because body image is formed from input from the vestibular, kinesthetic, proprioceptive, visual, and tactile systems, movement is an all-encompassing medium for the development of an individual's self-concept (Erfer, 1995).

Movement Analysis

Not only is dance/movement therapy unique because the primary modality for treatment is movement, but observation and assessment based on movement parameters are also key to the work of the field. Movement analysis is a broad and extremely complex field that allows dance/movement therapists to complete holistic movement observations of an individual's entire way of interacting with the world through movement. Dance/movement therapists use movement analysis to determine how people are relating, expressing, and experiencing on a nonverbal level, exemplifying Irmgard Bartenieff's theory that "inner connectivity breeds outer expressivity" (Hackney, 2002, p. 34). Dance/ movement therapists also use movement analysis to plan and guide their therapeutic interventions, consequently increasing emotional connectedness for individuals who struggle to unify their inner and outer selves. Additionally, dance/movement therapists may also use movement analysis to identify movement deficits in order to improve functional movement skills.

There are several different systems for movement assessment, but one widely used system is Laban Movement Analysis. In the early 1900s, Rudolf Laban began laying the groundwork for what would eventually become the comprehensive system of Laban Movement Analysis (Levy, 2005; Newlove & Dalby, 2004). In the 1950s, Laban's work was incorporated for therapeutic use by English dance therapists. Once integrated, the system provided a language for therapists who were looking to describe patient movement in an accessible format (Levy, 2005).

As it is known today, Laban Movement Analysis (LMA) is a complex system used to observe, describe, notate, and understand movement patterns. This is a complex, multifaceted system that allows an observer to understand the subtle characteristics and intention that define a movement. Because of its complexity, we only discuss a few elements of the system in this chapter. The first is Laban's Basic Efforts. The Basic Efforts have four categories, each defined by two polarities. These eight different elements allow us to understand a person's attitude toward each of the four main qualitative elements: *space* (directing or indirecting), *weight* (strong weight/increasing pressure or light weight/decreasing pressure), *time* (quickness or sustainment), and *flow* (binding or freeing). In addition to the Basic Efforts, the categories of space, weight, and time combine to form Action Drives, descriptively named *float*, *punch*, *glide*, *slash*, *dab*, *wring*, *flick*, and *press* (Newlove & Dalby, 2004).

Another element of the system is Body, emphasizing the patterns and tendencies of a person's body in motion. In this area especially, Irmgard Bartenieff made great contributions in the application of LMA to the field of dance/movement therapy (Bartenieff & Lewis, 1980; Levy, 2005). Bartenieff, a dancer and physical therapist, combined concepts from both LMA and physical therapy to create her own approach to movement. Bartenieff stressed the importance of viewing movement as a complex, interrelated whole, and she implored clinicians to look at an individual's total movement profile while emphasizing their potential movement expression. She also cautioned therapists away from pointing out a client's movement deficits, but rather engaging the client nonverbally in activities that would draw out any diminished movement (Levy, 2005). As Bartenieff saw it, the therapist was responsible for "finding the correct activities that supported the development of specific muscle systems, which, in turn, affected certain emotional attitudes" (as cited in Levy, 2005, p. 115).

Out of Bartenieff's movement system (Bartenieff Fundamentals) and the ongoing work of certified movement analysts evolved the Patterns of Total Body Connectivity, which "form the basis for our patterns of relationship and connection as we live our embodied lives; they provide models for our connectedness" (Hackney, 2002, p. 13). Each Pattern of Total Body Connectivity represents a specific level of human development and experience, in addition to a relational component. The six patterns progress developmentally, beginning with Breath and Progressing toward the final *Cross-Lateral* connectivity. The goal in the realization of all six Patterns of Total Body Connectivity is that through them individuals will experience lively interplay between their inner and outer selves, with "inner connectivity breeding outer expressivity" (Hackney, 2002, p. 34). In other words, increasing people's functional movement skills will eventually allow them a greater range for and capability of personal expressivity.

Assumptions about the underlying tenets of movement rest at the foundation of the body connectivities. The first tenet is the understanding that as we move we change, and change is thus fundamental. The second understanding is that relationship and connection are also fundamental—by moving and changing in relationship to others, we experience our embodied selves. Third is the underlying assumption that a patterning of body connections is fundamental; people will develop certain preferences and patterns that dictate how they move and thus relate to the world (Hackney, 2002).

I have found that these six developmental movement patterns are essential to my work with children, as they are naturally integrating and accessible for clients. The first pattern is *Breath*, which provides the foundation and grounding for all patterns that follow. Breath can be observed and brought to conscious awareness using a variety of breathing techniques and activities. When working with children, imagery plays a large role in building breath support. Examples of this may include providing a visual of a balloon and then practicing blowing up that balloon, pretending to blow out candles on a birthday cake, or flapping one's arms to fly while inhaling (arms up) and exhaling (arms down) in connection with the flapping motions.

The second pattern is the *Core-Distal* connectivity, described psychologically by Hackney (2002): "Before I can confidently move on my own in the world, I need to have a sense of my own center" (p. 67). This pattern of connectivity begins at the center, or core, of the body and radiates all the way out to the distal ends of the extremities. Movement from distal to core implies an ability to process and internalize the self in relationship to a newly discovered other, or outer (Hackney, 2002). Psychologically, Core-Distal is symbolic of an individual's ability to individuate and integrate, bringing his or her many moveable parts back to the core.

Moving on, the next pattern is the *Head-Tail* connectivity. This is an important connection because our head and tail are in ever-changing, constant relationship through the connection of our spine. People with strong Head-Tail connectivities feel confident in how to carry and move their bodies in the world, proclaiming a sense of "this is who I am."

When individuals move on to develop their *Upper-Lower* connectivity, they are beginning to differentiate in their bodies, understanding that some parts of the body fulfill certain functions and others fulfill different functions (e.g., walking with my lower body and writing with my upper body). Some psychological implications of understanding the Upper-Lower connection include knowing how to support ourselves, the ability to push away and set boundaries, standing on our own two feet, and claiming personal power (Hackney, 2002).

Next comes the *Body-Half* connectivity, where the Upper-Lower connection unites and instead the body splits into sidedness—right and left sides. This splitting into right and left underlies our brain patterning in sidedness or handedness. Functionally speaking, one side of the body practices stability and the other mobility, while psychologically this splitting is related to our ability to clarify, evaluate, and make decisions.

The final connectivity, *Cross-Lateral* connectivity, is the last to develop and the most complex pattern. The Cross-Lateral connectivity looks at the body in quadrants and examines the diagonal connection of the body (e.g., the connection between the right upper body and left lower body). Hackney (2002) refers to this final phase of differentiation as the "zenith of early childhood movement skills" (p. 198). When children learn to crawl, they begin in a Body-Half "army crawl" (right arm moving with right leg) and then develop to crawling Cross-Laterally (right arm and left leg forward). The achievement of the Cross-Lateral connection symbolizes integration, connecting the whole body with all parts in relationship (Hackney, 2002).

This basic understanding of Laban Movement Analysis and the Patterns of Total Body Connectivity will be helpful as we move on to the case studies, where these assessment tools are discussed, along with the previously covered tenets of dance/movement therapy and general goals for working with children with developmental delays.

CASE STUDIES

Individual

Lila is a young girl with autism spectrum disorder. I met Lila at the age of 2 years and 4 months, shortly following her initial diagnosis. At this point, Lila was entirely nonverbal and was learning to communicate using a few signs. She lacked imaginative and functional play skills and was easily distressed. Lila preferred to be with a few particular adults/ therapists, and she did not care for interacting with other children. She would begin crying at the onset of a day, and she would not be able to recover from this distress without long and recurrent periods of swinging.

Lila went through a lengthy period of adjustment at the onset of her intensive therapy (both group and individual) where she experienced distress and anxiety, evidenced by a great deal of crying and inability to remain with peers in the group setting. After working through this period, it became obvious that Lila loved movement and music. Lila was especially skilled at imitating movement, even when her imitation skills lacked in other areas (e.g., imitating ways to functionally play with an object or toy). Six months after she started treatment, I began doing group and individual dance/movement therapy with Lila. At this point, I also conducted a movement analysis on her. This analysis displayed Lila's preferential movement signature, and from this assessment, I was able to create specific movement goals for her.

At the time of the initial assessment, I observed that Lila's Core-Distal connection stood out the most when watching her movement, in particular her interesting and strong awareness of her distal ends (i.e., being fascinated by sign language song actions or watching her feet move by tapping her toes) while lacking the full connection between her distal parts and her core. Thus, Lila seemed to have a strong understanding of her distal parts—both hands and feet—without any awareness of or ability to connect these parts back into her core and the center of her body and self.

In addition to the relationship between her distal and core parts, Lila also lacked an Upper-Lower body connection. This was possibly most evident through her lack of homologous body awareness and motor skills. By her third birthday, Lila had not yet achieved the gross motor skills of either running or jumping with two feet, typically beginning to develop by the age of 24 months and fully developed by 36 months (World Health Organization, 2008). She would carefully observe peers jumping and try to mimic their movement with little ability to motor plan and yield-push her body into the floor in order to reach and pull her body into a jump.

At this point, Lila's inability to jump was possibly connected to the lack of time she spent exploring the weight efforts of light and strong weight (part of Laban's Basic Efforts). Lila had a preference for the space effort and would spend a great deal of her time observing others using space efforts, both indirecting and directing. Although she was found to be mostly residing in and focusing on her relationship to space, Lila spent little time paying attention to her relationship with weight (e.g., her ability to use her own weight to press into and then off of the floor in a jump). Additionally, Lila advanced forward in space by leading from her torso or midsection, with what looked like little awareness for the functionality of using her lower body in order to mobilize (part of her lacking understanding of her Upper-Lower connection).

With these observations and others in mind, movement goals were created for Lila. Her initial goals focused on increasing her awareness of both the Core-Distal connection (specifically her core) and the homologous movement related to the Upper-Lower connectivity. Following the first observation, Lila participated in group dance/movement therapy two times per week for one-hour increments. During these sessions, a variety of interventions and modalities encouraged Lila to explore movement in her goal areas.

In her dance/movement therapy groups, as part of the initial body warm-up, Lila completed a warm-up that was structured using animal movements that activated the six Patterns of Total Body Connectivity in a developmental progression. The warm-up moved through the six connectivities, from Breath to Cross-Lateral, assigning an animal to each connectivity—doing the movement for each animal allowed the group members (including Lila) to locate and experience each of the connections (e.g., making a giant starfish for the Core-Distal connection and swimming like a fish on her belly, first arms then legs and then both together to experience the Upper-Lower connection).

Helping Lila to build her body awareness also led to her further integration and development. Utilizing Marian Chace's emphasis on and concept around *body action*, Lila increased her own body awareness. Each day in dance/movement therapy she would first "find" and touch her knees, and then practice bending her knees, eventually leading to a full body bounce. At first this was done with some assistance from me, but eventually Lila was able to locate and move her body on her own. With this new awareness and ability to activate her lower body, Lila was able to conceptualize and then physicalize the motor planning necessary to bend her knees to yield into the ground and then push off into either a run or jump.

Lastly, Lila grew to love yoga, and the integration of yoga poses into her dance/movement therapy routine allowed her to visualize and integrate diversified movement concepts. This allowed Lila to increase and diversify her movement repertoire. Lila, who was both visually and kinesthetically astute, was able to look at a picture of a yoga pose and then manipulate her body into that pose independently. Poses such as "cow" and "cat" in an oscillating pattern helped Lila to locate and activate the core of her body.

Six months after the initial assessment, a second movement observation was conducted. The analysis showed that Lila had made significant strides in these movement goal areas. By month 3 she was running and jumping, first with physical support (i.e., holding hands to run or hands on the knees to show her where to bend before a jump) and then entirely independently. By month 6 Lila was integrating yielding movement throughout her whole body. In learning to yield into the ground, Lila was increasing her relationship to the weight effort, and her ability to yield was beginning to give her freedom of movement in her hips, which had been bound (or tight) before and hindered her ability to explore her Upper-Lower connectivity. Lila's twisting and free-flow movement, as well as connection to her breath support, indicated her growing sense of contentment with her environment. In addition to these movement developments, Lila progressed quickly in many other areas during the 6-month period. Most notably, she went from being almost entirely nonverbal to blossoming and communicating primarily through verbalizations. Thus, Lila's communication development exemplified Bartenieff's theory that inner connectivity breeds outer expressivity (Bartenieff & Lewis, 1980).

Girls' Group

In the previous case study, my goal was to explain how a dance/movement therapist sets and carries out movement goals for an individual. In contrast, this group example focuses less on movement analysis and goal setting and more on the structure of a dance/movement therapy group following the Chacian format.

The session described as follows was the 12th in a series of 18 sessions held at an outpatient clinic. The group described was a voluntary group that met on a weekly basis. The group was designed for teen girls, and on this particular week was composed of four females between the ages of 12 and 15 years old, myself, and a mental health co-therapist. The participants were all diagnosed with some form of autism spectrum disorder, and each had at least one other diagnosis in addition (including reactive attachment disorder, posttraumatic stress disorder from preadoptive trauma, and Down syndrome).

Each member of the group had a specialized treatment plan. In addition to individual goals, overarching group goals influenced the guiding interventions in each session. The first goal was that group members would *increase their sense of self by fostering body awareness and nurturing their individual self-concept.* The teens in this group appeared to lack a solid sense of self. This was evident in movement by concave postures, an inability to access sinking and rising in their vertical planes (if present, this is psychologically indicative of a strong sense of self), and lack of physical (and emotional) boundaries. Thus, this group was meant as a safe place for group members to explore and foster their personal sense of self while in an accepting environment. This often happened in the group through movement exploration and affirmation (e.g., excitedly cheering each other on in vertical posture and with energized movement).

Secondly, group members were challenged to *increase interpersonal communication skills.* Specifically, group members were asked to negotiate conflicts in a prosocial manner within the group setting. In the dance/movement therapy setting, the group members learned about and practiced skills related to reading nonverbal cues (e.g., facial expression or posture), a skill that is often very difficult for adolescents with autism spectrum disorders. They also participated in group rhythmic activity/movement, practiced moving using direct space (to kinesthetically experience both asking questions and stating comments directly), and developed their use of eye contact and safe spatial boundaries (not too close but near enough to get someone's attention) when relating to others in the group.

Lastly, group members worked to *increase their ability to relate to and understand the feelings and experiences of others*. In this particular grouping, all of the group members struggled with empathy—they were highly aware of and sensitive to actions by others that hurt their own feelings, but they lacked the ability to comprehend the impact of their actions on others. In verbal interactions, the impact made by other's comments is physically evident in the full-bodied postural responses to both negative and positive feedback from peers. Thus, we regularly practiced reflecting and mirroring the movement of peers in order to begin the process of kinesthetically attuning to others.

With these goals in mind, following is the outline of one specific session. The group typically began by sitting in a circle (marked with colored rubber spots on the floor) for a brief check-in followed by body warm-up. One group member struggled with needing her own space and typically requested to remove her colored sitting spot away from the circle in order to have more personal space (a skill in itself that we worked on mastering for nearly one year). On this day, this member was the first to arrive, and she followed her weekly ritual of moving her favorite red spot away from the circle and toward the wall. Once she was seated, the second and third members entered the room. For the first time, the two members independently noticed and asked the peer if they could move the entire circle toward her spot at the wall, which she agreed to. At this point, group members began laughing and making silly jokes together, and the fourth member entered the group. Meeting them at this place, I suggested one minute of complete silliness before moving on to the warm-up. Group members accepted this proposal and seemed to enjoy the chance to be silly and laugh in each other's company. At the end of the minute, the girls were able to shift their focus following a prompt (when working with this particular group, prompts and foreshadows, e.g., stating "We have one minute" were extremely helpful for creating smooth transitions).

Following this minute, the group stood up, the music was started, and members began moving. Because the energy that day appeared to be silly, I began by continuing their exploration of silly through movement. Then one group member requested a chance to lead a movement and have the others follow (something we did often in order to increase opportunities for mirroring). Other group members also requested chances to lead or dance on their own. As a response to this apparent interest in having a chance to shine, as well as a natural transition for the group from the body warm-up to the theme development and exploration portion of the session, I suggested making a stage space out of our colored floor spots and giving each member 1 minute to dance and perform for the others. The group responded with unanimous favor to this idea (evident by vertical postural movement and fervent head nodding), and followed through with the idea, supporting each other by clapping in synchrony and cheering during their peers' turns (naturally creating rhythmic group activity). This was followed by a brief verbal check-in regarding their personal feelings and preferences to lead/perform or follow/watch within the group.

Next, a different group member requested making the stage into a room-length runway, a similar activity we had done in the past in which each member could dance down the runway with group members on either side watching and cheering on. In an attempt to expand on this idea, I suggested that instead of a single-person runway, we would begin this week by dancing the runway in pairs (another opportunity to practice communication through movement). This concept developed thematically with several purposeful movement interventions. First, the group practiced reflecting and matching their partners while moving down the runway simultaneously and finding ways to dance together. Next, I gave an intervention to move in slow motion, knowing that moving in sustained, or slow, time was typically difficult for this group of clients. Third, the group followed an intervention to move while staying close to the floor/using low space (an attempt to expand their use of kinespheric reach space and general dimension of orientation). Lastly, I suggested moving down the runway pretending to be feathers (accessing light weight and free flow, from Laban's Basic Efforts). In this final intervention, one pair was struggling with the movement concept, and I suggested that the first pair serve as wind for the feathers. This prompt helped bring attention to their breathing and also motivated the reluctant pair. The intervention resulted in all group members moving in synchrony until it was time for the group to end. The group ended with minimal verbal processing, but group members participated in an ending good-bye ritual before putting on their shoes and leaving the group room.

This example demonstrates the use of the broad structure of the group, including a body warm-up, theme development and exploration, and verbal processing and closure. In addition, this example further demonstrates the integration of movement analysis and movement-based goals and interventions, resulting in a full-length group in which movement was the primary modality.

CONCLUSION

As this chapter concludes, my hope is that the background information, theory, techniques, and case studies have given you some insight into the unique field of dance/movement therapy. Moreover, I hope that beyond the theory and practice, you have been given examples that illustrate the power of movement as both a language and a therapeutic vehicle. This chapter has only skimmed the possibilities available when bringing movement into the lives of children. Reading the movements, or nonverbal language, of each individual child enables therapists to better understand and attune to the child's emotions and needs. Beyond dance/movement therapy, an awareness of children's movement informs *any* therapist working with children. The movement has the power to speak for itself.

SPECIALIZED TRAINING AND RESOURCES

Training and Certification

In order to practice as dance/movement therapists, individuals must have obtained Master's-level training in an approved program of the American Dance Therapy Association. The approved dance/movement therapy programs cover a range of information, including training in both counseling and dance/movement therapy, in addition to 700 hours of clinical fieldwork and internships. Upon graduating from an approved program, dance/movement therapists receive the level of Registered Dance/Movement Therapist (R-DMT). Achieving the second level of competence for the field, Board Certified Dance/Movement Therapist (BC-DMT), indicates that an individual has been approved for this second level by the BC-DMT credentialing board following several years of work in the field, supervision, and a rigorous application process. BC-DMTs are prepared to provide supervision and training in the field, as well as to work in private practice. For more information on the education and training requirements for dance/movement therapists, consult the national organization website at www.adta.org

Professional Organization

The American Dance Therapy Association (ADTA) was founded in 1966 and is the only professional organization in the United States for dance/movement therapists. In its dedication to the profession, the ADTA holds an annual conference for education and training, and also supports the efforts of state and regional chapters in these areas. The ADTA also publishes the *American Journal of Dance Therapy* and a national newsletter, in addition to promoting the field through other avenues of social media. Thirdly, the ADTA advocates for the development and expansion of the field of dance/movement therapy on both national and international levels. To learn more about the ADTA, visit their website at www.adta.org

Ethics

The ADTA has a Code of Ethics to which members and credentialed dance/movement therapist are required to adhere. The Code defines rules of conduct for dance/movement therapists, as well as responsible, professional behavior for those working in the field. In addition to the Code of Ethics, dance/movement therapists adhere to the ADTA Standards of Ethical Practice, or specific guidelines that serve as a model for dance/movement therapists in practice.

Further Resources

If you are interested in learning more about the field of dance/movement therapy, consider subscribing to the *American Journal of Dance Therapy*, which is published biannually. In addition, a wealth of resources are available on the national organization website at www.adta.org where you can watch videos and view slideshows of dance/movement therapy in action. The website has links to general articles about the field, and resources are broken down by population and illness, for those who are looking for something in particular.

List of Terms

Attunement A dance/movement therapy technique used to build a sense of empathy between therapist and client. Attunement is achieved by sharing qualities of muscle tension when relating on a nonverbal level (Loman, 1995).

Dance/Movement Therapy As defined by the American Dance Therapy Association, dance/movement therapy is the "psychotherapeutic use of movement as a process which furthers the emotional, social, cognitive and physical integration of the individual" (American Dance Therapy Association, 2008). Dance/movement therapists examine both the experience of moving and the significance of that experience for the mover. The dance/movement therapist is specially trained to observe the client's movement patterns as "expressions of the intrapsychic, interpersonal, intersubjective and cultural realms of experiencing" (Mason, unpublished paper, p. 7).

Laban Movement Analysis Laban Movement Analysis (LMA) is a complex system used to observe, describe, notate, and understand movement patterns. The system was devised by Rudolf Laban and is widely used, especially in the field of dance/ movement therapy (Newlove & Dalby, 2004).

Patterns of Total Body Connectivity The concept of the six connectivities was originally introduced by Rudolf Laban and later further developed by both Irmgard Bartenieff and Peggy Hackney. These connectivities consist of breath, core-distal, head-tail, upper-lower, body-half, and cross-lateral. When working together in an integrated fashion, the six connectivities are believed to indicate both internal and external harmony. This harmony is also contingent on the belief that a sense of stability is necessary for mobility, and mobility is needed in order to achieve stability (Hackney, 2002).

REFERENCES

Adler, J. (2003). From autism to the discipline of authentic movement. *American Journal of Dance Therapy, 25*(1), 5–16.

American Dance Therapy Association. (2008). Retrieved from www.adta.org/about/factsheet.cfm

Bartenieff, I., & Lewis, D. (1980). *Body movement: Coping with the environment.* New York, NY: Gordon and Breach.

Berrol, C. (2006). Neuroscience meets dance/movement therapy: Mirror neurons, the therapeutic process and empathy. *The Arts in Psychotherapy, 33,* 302–315.

Canner, N. (1968). . . . *And a time to dance.* Boston, MA: Beacon Press.

Capello, P. (2008). Dance/movement therapy with children throughout the world. *American Journal of Dance Therapy, 30,* 24–36.

Chaiklin, S., & Schmais, C. (1993). The Chace approach to dance therapy. In S. Sandel, S. Chaiklin, & A. Lohn (Eds.), *Foundations of dance/movement therapy: The life and work of Marian Chace* (pp. 75–97). Columbia, MD: The Marian Chase Memorial Fund of the American Dance Therapy Association.

Erfer, T. (1995). Treating children with autism in a public school system. In F. J. Levy, J. P. Fried, & F. Leventhal (Eds.), *Dance and other expressive arts therapies* (pp. 191–211). New York, NY: Routledge.

Hackney, P. (2002). *Making connections: Total body integration through Bartenieff fundamentals.* New York, NY: Routledge.

Kestenberg, J. A., Loman, S., Lewis, P., & Sossin, K. M. (1999). *The meaning of movement: Developmental and clinical perspectives of the Kestenberg Movement Profile.* New York, NY: Brunner-Routledge.

Levy, F. (2005). *Dance movement therapy: A healing art.* Reston, VA: National Dance Association.

Loman, S. (1995). The case of Warren: A KMP approach to autism. In F. J. Levy, J. P. Fried, & F. Leventhal (Eds.), *Dance and other expressive arts therapies: When words are not enough* (pp. 213–224). New York, NY: Routledge.

Mason, M. (n.d.) *The process of change from a self-psychological perspective.* Unpublished manuscript, Columbia College, Chicago, IL.

Meekums, B. (2002). *Dance movement therapy: A creative psychotherapeutic approach.* London, England: Sage.

Newlove, J., & Dalby, J. (2004). *Laban for all.* New York, NY: Routledge.

Thom, L. (2010). From simple line to expressive movement: The use of creative movement to enhance socio-emotional development in the preschool curriculum. *American Journal of Dance Therapy, 32,* 100–112.

Wolf-Schein, E., Fisch, G., & Cohen, I. (1985). A study of the use of nonverbal systems in the differential diagnosis of autistic, mentally retarded and Fragile X individuals. *American Journal of Dance Therapy, 8,* 67–80.

World Health Organization. (2008). Retrieved from www.who.int/childgrowth/standards/motor_milestones/en/index.html

7

Music Therapy

Susan Hadley and Nicole Steele

INTRODUCTION

Music is very important in the lives and development of children (Kemple, Batey, & Hartle, 2004). It encourages creativity and exploration. It provides a nonverbal means of communication, when words may be difficult or inadequate. Music can reduce stress and anxiety. It stimulates language and movement. It can be used to develop listening and social skills and also to develop cognitive skills. It can help to build confidence and to foster relationships with others. And it is fun and aesthetically fulfilling. Thus, music contributes to the cognitive, physical, social, and emotional well-being of children of all ages. Music is a medium of play.

Play, like music, is very important in the lives and development of children. According to Ginsberg (2007), "Play allows children to use their creativity while developing their imagination, dexterity, and physical, cognitive, and emotional strength" (p. 183). Thus, the blending of play therapy and the expressive art of music produces a powerful way to reach children and effect lasting change. Music therapists utilize these principles when working with children to meet their cognitive, physical, social, emotional, and behavioral needs. Although they are not trained in the therapeutic benefits of music, and perhaps do not possess the same musical abilities as music therapists, play therapists can also incorporate music into their approach with children to meet the same needs.

Overview of Research

In addition to anecdotal reports on the effectiveness of music therapy, music therapists have a long history of research in music therapy that has documented the effectiveness of the use of music in clinical practice. There is a wide variety of approaches to music therapy research from both positivist and nonpositivist paradigms (Wheeler, 2005). However, in line with health professionals in many international contexts, in 2005 the American Music Therapy Association developed its *"Research Strategic Priority*, with one of its central purposes being to advance the music therapy field through research promoting the *Evidence-Based Practice* (EBP) of music therapy" (Abrams, 2010, p. 351). Thus, in recent years in the United States, there has been a rise in meta-analyses and systematic reviews on music therapy research.

Pediatric Medical Setting

Standley and Whipple (2003) conducted a meta-analysis on 29 empirical research studies that compared music and no-music conditions during medical treatment of pediatric patients. The overall results of this meta-analysis were that (a) the use of music is significantly better than no music in pediatric medical treatment; (b) actively engaging patients in musical experiences is better than passive listening; (c) the use of live music is better than recorded music; (d) the use of music has greater effect for people having noninvasive and major invasive procedures than for minor invasive procedures; (e) the greatest effects are achieved for adolescents, then infants, with lesser effects found for children between the ages of 4 and 12; and (f) behavioral observation of pain and distress reveal modest effect sizes in comparison to physiological measures and self-reports of pain and distress. Other findings were that there were no differentiated effects related to who selected the music (i.e., whether the patient, the music therapist, or the medical personnel selected the music), and that there were no differentiated effects related to gender (p. 11).

Similarly, Klassen, Liang, Tjosvold, Klassen, and Hartling (2008) conducted a systematic review of 19 randomized controlled trials to examine the efficacy of music therapy on pain and anxiety in children undergoing medical procedures. Although the methodological quality of the included studies was generally poor, the overall results of the review demonstrated that music therapy significantly reduced anxiety and pain in children undergoing medical and dental procedures.

Examining the effectiveness of music interventions on psychological and physiological responses in patients with coronary heart disease, Bradt and Dileo (2009) conducted a systematic review of 23 randomized controlled trials. Most of the studies they included examined the effects of listening to prerecorded music rather than music offered by trained music therapists. The findings suggested that music listening may have a beneficial effect on blood pressure and heart rate in people with coronary heart disease and may reduce anxiety in myocardial infarction patients. Music listening may also reduce pain and respiratory rate, but the effect size was small and the quality of evidence was not strong.

In a similar systematic review of seven randomized and quasirandomized controlled trials, Bradt, Magee, Dileo, Wheeler, and McGilloway (2010) examined the effects of music therapy with standard care versus standard care alone or standard care combined with other therapies as a rehabilitation intervention with people with acquired brain injury. The overall results of the review suggested that rhythmic auditory stimulation may be beneficial for improving the measure of walking. Given the paucity of information in the included studies, they were unable to examine the effect of music therapy on other outcomes.

Examining the effect of music interventions on the psychological and physical outcomes of people with cancer, Bradt, Dileo, Grocke, and Magill (2011) reviewed 30 randomized controlled trials and quasirandomized trials. They found that most of the trials were at high risk of bias and, therefore, the results need to be interpreted with caution, but the findings suggested that music therapy and music medicine interventions may have a beneficial effect on anxiety, pain, mood, quality of life, heart rate, respiratory rate, and blood pressure for cancer patients.

Pediatric Behavioral and Mental Health

Gold, Voracek, and Wigram (2004) conducted a meta-analysis on 11 empirical research studies to examine the effects of music therapy for children and adolescents with psychopathology. The overall results of this meta-analysis were that the effects of music therapy tended to be greater for people with behavioral and developmental disorders than for those with emotional disorders. Music therapy effects tended to be greater when using humanistic, psychodynamic, and eclectic approaches than when using behavioral approaches. Furthermore, the effects of music therapy tended to be greater for behavioral and developmental outcomes than for social skills and self-concept. Examining the effectiveness of music therapy to reduce the symptoms of depression in particular, Maratos, Gold, Wang, and Crawford (2008) conducted a systematic review of five empirical studies. Because of marked variations in the interventions offered, the populations studied, and the outcome measures used, quantitative data synthesis and meta-analysis were not appropriate. Findings from four of the studies did indicate greater reductions in symptoms of depression among those in the music therapy treatment groups, suggesting that music therapy is a feasible treatment approach for people with depression. However, the authors concluded that more empirical studies need to be conducted in this area.

Also in the area of mental health, Pelletier (2004) conducted a meta-analysis on 22 quantitative studies to examine the effect of music on decreasing arousal caused by stress. The overall results of the meta-analysis were that music alone and music-assisted relaxation techniques significantly decreased arousal, and that the amount of stress reduction was significantly different when considering age, type of stress, type of intervention, music-assisted relaxation technique, musical preference, and previous music experience.

Focusing on adolescents, McFerran (2010) conducted a systematic review of five decades of music therapy literature. She noted that the majority of music therapy work with adolescents takes place in institutions such as hospitals, inpatient mental health institutions, residential settings, or hospices. In terms of theoretical orientation, psychodynamic was the most commonly adopted approach, followed by humanistic. Behavioral approaches were less commonly adopted by music therapists working with adolescents. The most commonly used music therapy methods with adolescents were live singing of songs, improvisation, and listening to and discussing prerecorded music. Music and movement and musical games were less frequently documented. In terms of the types of challenges faced by adolescent clients in music therapy, McFerran found that nearly 40% of those described had a mental illness or a major medical illness, 31% were diagnosed with a disability, 25% had emotional and behavioral problems, and 21% were classified as at-risk. The major goals addressed with this population were identity formation and social goals, with 56% of articles noting these as goals.

Implications of Research for Music Therapy and Play Therapy

In the previously cited research, it is indicated that actively engaging people in musical experiences facilitated by a music therapist tends to yield greater effects than when music is listened to passively or administered by a nonspecialist. However, even music facilitated by a nonspecialist was seen to yield positive results. As such, there is support for the *careful* use of music by nonspecialists.

In order to blend music with play therapy, it is important to explore how the two fields overlap. According to the Association for Play Therapy (2013), play therapy involves "the systematic use of a theoretical model to establish an interpersonal process wherein trained play therapists use the therapeutic powers of play to help clients prevent or resolve psychosocial difficulties and achieve optimal growth and development." Although music therapists also address physical and cognitive needs in addition to psychological, social, and emotional needs, there are important overlaps. In both music and play therapies, our mediums are used as vehicles for self-expression, communication, socialization, and recreation. Both can be educational and enjoyable, and both are integral in a child's life.

MUSIC THERAPY: PROCESS AND PROCEDURES

Music therapy is a diverse discipline, practiced in many cultural contexts around the world, from a variety of theoretical orientations. Given this diversity, music therapy has been defined in many ways, each nuanced to capture the context in which the particular way of practicing music therapy was developed. For example, the American Music Therapy Association (AMTA; 2013) defines it as follows:

> Music Therapy is the clinical and evidence-based use of music interventions to accomplish individualized goals within a therapeutic relationship by a credentialed professional who has completed an approved music therapy program.

This definition clearly situates music therapy as a clinical practice based on research evidence and emphasizes that it involves specialized training through approved programs. The AMTA (2013) goes on to state:

> Music Therapy is an established health profession in which music is used within a therapeutic relationship to address physical, emotional, cognitive, and social needs of individuals.

Although there is no universally accepted, all-encompassing definition of music therapy, Bruscia (1998) developed a working definition that attempts to synthesize various definitions of music therapy found in the literature over decades:

> Music therapy is a systematic process of intervention wherein the therapist helps the client to promote health, using music experiences, and the relationships that develop through them as dynamic forces of change. (p. 20)

In this definition, Bruscia emphasizes the systematic process of assessment, treatment, and evaluation, which music therapists employ, and the dynamic nature of the interrelationships between the client and the music, the client and the therapist, and the therapist and the music. As with the AMTA definition (2013), specialized training is also indicated in Bruscia's definition in terms of the music therapist's dual expertise in music and in the complex processes and dynamics that evolve in therapeutic contexts. Addressing this relationship, Bruscia (1998) notes that music therapy is transdisciplinary (p. 6) in nature, "at once an art, a science, and an interpersonal process" (p. 10).

MUSIC THERAPY METHODS

Music therapists use both live music and recorded music, depending on the needs and goals that are being addressed. Many music therapists advocate the use of live music because of both its acoustic properties and its greater potential for creative and flexible use. The musical experiences that music therapists engage in with clients include four distinct types: listening to music, performing music (that is, re-creating already composed music), composing music, and improvising music. Within each of these methods of engaging in music, a variety of different approaches may be used, each addressing different therapeutic aims. Music therapists do not prescribe certain types of music for certain conditions, but rather choose music and musical experiences based on a multitude of factors, including, but not limited to, the musical preferences of the client, the needs that are being addressed, the abilities and limitations of the client, and the context in which therapy is occurring.

Music Listening

Some of the types of music listening (receptive) experiences music therapists engage in with music therapy participants include music for relaxation; music and imagery; music biofeedback; music entrainment (to change physiological states such as heart rate, breathing rate); music for pain management; music and movement; music appreciation; music for reminiscence; and, listening to songs, discussing the meaning of the song's themes for the listener. Music therapists engage participants in listening experiences for a variety of reasons, such as to induce a relaxed state, to alter physiological states, to stimulate or organize movement, for aesthetic pleasure, to stimulate memories, to explore emotions, to stimulate social interactions, and more.

Case Study: Rose—Pediatric Oncology Unit

Rose was an 18-year-old patient who had just undergone a bone marrow transplant. When she was brought back to her hospital room, she asked for me to come and play some music. Prior to her transplant we had spent time singing together and discussing songs. When I went in, Rose was quite lethargic. She was in pain and feeling nauseous. I quickly surmised that actively engaging her in music was not appropriate. So, I asked her whether she would like me to play a little music on my guitar. She nodded. I wanted to play music that would be soothing for her. As I began to play, I was very conscious of a steady beeping sound coming from one of the machines. As a musician, I knew I needed to play in time with the beeping or it would produce more tension in her. So, I played at half the speed of the beeping sound (which I soon realized was her heart monitor). As I played and hummed, I noticed that her heart rate was quite elevated, at around 120 beats per minute. After a while I noticed that the heart rate had gone down to about 110 beats per minute. The music and the monitor seemed to be synchronized. I decided to test to see whether they were, because if they were, I could help Rose to relax further. I very slightly increased my speed of playing and noticed that her heart rate also slightly increased. So, I decided to very gradually reduce my speed over time. I played for her for about half an hour and had reduced her heart rate to 80 beats per minute, which I maintained for at least 10 minutes. When I left her she was sleeping. The next day, one of the nursing staff informed me that Rose reported that her experience during the music playing was that her nausea dissipated, her pain was lessened, and she felt more relaxed and able to sleep.

Case Study: Maria—Cardiac Intensive Care Unit

Maria was a 15-year-old girl with a severe heart disease who was actively listed on the heart transplant list when I met her. Her medical team consulted music therapy and child life as they expressed their concerns that she was becoming withdrawn and depressed. She was a fiery young lady with jet-black hair, collages of neon sneakers with the latest urban fashion, and a small Cuban flag on her wall. In our first session she wore her bright, large headphones around her neck, from which I could hear fast grooves of Cuban music pouring. Maria expressed that she had never played an instrument, but she had always loved music. In that session she talked about her home, her love of her mother's home-cooked Cuban classics like black beans and rice, friends, family, school, and eventually how "bored" she was of being stuck in the hospital. I asked her to share a few of her favorite songs with me, and she played me a variety of Cuban, Latin, and pop music as she closed her eyes, laid her head back, and nodded to the grooves. After building a rapport with her, we also spent time together playing drums and other percussion along to her favorite songs.

As Maria's hospitalization progressed, she became a bit weaker and would fatigue with simple daily tasks. On the days that she could not play, she would ask me to play the guitar, and she would often fall asleep as I played soft and slow melodic lines, some of which mimicked tracks she had played for me. After Maria received her heart transplant, we continued to share in music making and music listening together. I was consulted by the medical team to assist Maria during her first heart catheterization and biopsy by providing music for relaxation, as she would not receive general anesthesia for the procedure. I met up with Maria at her bedside to make a plan before her procedure. She requested that "you play that music that puts me to sleep because I gotta stay calm." The medical team created a space for me at the head of Maria's bed. She was draped in sterile attire, but she could see my eyes under the cap and mask and I could see hers. I continued to play soft and soothing music as she fell in and out of sleep. After a few more weeks in the hospital, Maria was discharged home. I continue to support her catheterizations and biopsies when she comes twice a year.

Music Performing

When music therapists engage participants in performing, or re-creating music that has already been composed, the experiences primarily include singing or playing instruments. Again, many varying needs may be met through engagement in singing or playing instruments, including increasing lung capacity, expressing or connecting with emotions, elevating mood states, developing motor coordination, improving range of motion, developing sensorimotor skills, developing cognitive skills, improving attention, addressing social skills, meeting spiritual needs, and so on.

Case Study: Sam—Pediatric Burns Unit

Sam was a 4-year-old boy who was admitted to the hospital because of severe burns to 85% of his body. He had been caught playing with matches, so his mother locked him in his bedroom. She did not, however, take the matches from him before putting him in his room. As a result, he continued to play with the matches. When I first met Sam, he was bandaged from head to foot, with just parts of his face and neck exposed. He was in extraordinary pain much of the time. When I came in with music, his eyes lit up. He had an obvious affinity with music. After a few sessions, while I was singing familiar children's songs with him, he would reach out to my guitar with his bandaged feet and strum the strings. He really loved doing this. Although his hands had been amputated, he would strum the guitar with the end of his arms as well. When the physical therapist saw this she was amazed, because Sam screamed out in pain whenever they tried to get him to move any part of his body. So, after discussing his needs and his positive relationship with music, we decided to collaborate. It was obvious that his desire to play music was in many ways distracting him from the pain he usually experienced in physical therapy.

With that knowledge, and the aim to have him cross his midline, we adapted some instruments for him to play. We took a pair of small hand cymbals and attached a Velcro strap on each one. We tied one around his arm just above his wrist. I took the other and placed it close enough for him to crash the cymbals as we sang his favorite songs. While he was hitting the cymbal, I would very gradually move my cymbal closer to his midline. Each time he would reach farther than the time before. We alternated sides frequently, strapping the cymbal on his right arm for one song and on his left for the next. Within weeks he was crossing his midline. Seeing these results, I continued to collaborate with the physical therapist to increase more motor skills (while addressing emotional needs and increasing lung capacity). After about six months we were all incredibly excited to see Sam take his first steps.

Case Study: Katie—Pediatric Intensive Care Unit

Katie was a 16-year-old girl diagnosed with Guillain-Barré syndrome, which caused her to have almost no movement or control of her arms or legs. Katie had spent most of her life prior to her illnesses (starting her hospitalizations with numerous gastrointestinal issues/infections progressing to Guillain-Barré) as an active teenager who was involved in chorus (achieving an honor's competition award the prior year), church, and horseback riding. I received a consult to see Katie from her primary doctor, as she was concerned that Katie was becoming depressed, the more she was unable to do the things she had once loved. Staff at the hospital had noticed that Katie was keeping the lights off more during the day and did not speak much to anyone. Katie was now dependent on people to assist her with almost every task of daily living.

In our first session, Katie was welcoming and briefly talked about her love of music, horses, God, and people. Katie's favorite music was mostly country and contemporary Christian. Katie reported she was tired after talking, but she requested that I played a few songs before I left. As I played the requested music, Katie closed her eyes, and a few tears came down her face. When the song ended, I asked if there was anything she needed. "Just wipe my tears and keep singing and playing," she said with a smile. I continued playing a few more songs and ended with a slow guitar song, as she fell asleep.

I continued to see Katie numerous times per week, and each time she requested songs to hear but did not participate in singing. During the sixth session, while I was singing the chorus of a song she requested every session, she started singing loudly along with me. She looked up to meet my eyes when the song was through and said, "I just felt ready to sing again." From that session on, Katie sang almost every word of every song we did together. She began inviting her nurses and doctors in to listen, and eventually we made recordings, which she took with her when she was discharged from the hospital to a rehabilitation facility.

Music Composition

Compositional experiences that music therapists engage in with music therapy participants include songwriting, lyric writing, writing instrumental pieces, creating music videos, and so on. These compositions may range from very simple to very complex. In this kind of experience, the participant is involved in communicating ideas, expressing emotions, making decisions, and utilizing creative potential. The end result is a product that can then be listened to or performed again and again, for one's own pleasure or to be shared with others. Songwriting and other compositional methods can bring a sense of mastery, enhance self-esteem, improve coping, and enhance social interaction.

Case Study: Janie—Pediatric Orthopedic Unit

Janie was an 11-year-old girl who had been admitted to the hospital after being hit by a car. When I first met Janie, she had both legs in traction. She told me that she wanted to learn the guitar while she was in the hospital. Given that she was going to be staying for quite some time, this seemed like a good choice. However, when I brought her a guitar to start learning on, she began asking me what other musical things kids in the hospital were doing. I mentioned all of the different ways in which music therapists work with patients. At the mention of songwriting, her eyes lit up. She told me with great excitement that she loved to write poetry.

The next time I visited, she had a book of poetry she wanted to share with me. Given her strong interest in writing poetry, we decided to try songwriting. She proceeded to quiz me on what other kids in the hospital were writing songs about. I told her it could be on anything at all, but she insisted that I provide her with examples. I mentioned that some patients wrote about what they miss at home, or about what they miss at school, or about their pets, or discussed their experiences inside the hospital. She launched into a song that described her accident and her experiences in the hospital. We created original lyrics, an original melody, and an original accompaniment. Her lyrics began with, "The first thing I remember I was being dragged across the street. My friends were all hysterical—I didn't know why that was. The next thing I knew, a stretcher was by my side. My friends were all there watching and my Dad was holding my hand." It was a long song with several verses, chronicling her entire experience. When we finished it, I asked whether she would like us to record it so that she would have a copy of it to listen to whenever she wanted.

While I was packing up after one session, Janie asked whether I could work with her friend, Katie, because she was feeling a lot of guilt. Katie had called Janie across the street just before Janie was hit by the car. Janie felt that music therapy might help Katie deal with her feelings. A few days later, a woman stopped me in the hallway and asked if I was the music therapist. After I confirmed that I was, she explained that she was Janie's mother, and she wanted to talk with me. She explained to me that Janie had shared her song with her family. I was pleased, but I did not think much of it until her mother explained that this was the first time since her accident that Janie had mentioned anything at all about the accident. The song had allowed her to let them know what she had gone through, and after that she was able to open up and talk with them about it.

Case Study: Kara—General Medical Unit

Most teenagers who have a love for hip-hop culture think they can write a rap song. The themes in rap songs deal with alienation or a sense of being wronged, so it is no coincidence that teens with various medical conditions relate so much to the genre. Kara was one of them. Kara had Gardner's syndrome, a disorder characterized by polyps and tumors in and on the colon. She was physically abused as a child, expediting the progress of her disease to the point where she had to undergo a complete enterectomy—her intestines had to be removed. Her father died of the same disease, her mother was often absent, and her sister was also hospitalized.

In one session, we were listening to "Just Fine," one of the most positive songs by Mary J. Blige, with a chorus that reinforces "my life's just fine, fine, fine. . . ." It's very upbeat, but the song also provides the opportunity to talk. "So I like what I see when I'm looking at me/When I'm walking past the mirror." I asked Kara how she felt about what she saw when she walked past the mirror. The song continues with the line, "You see I wouldn't change my life/My life's just fine, fine, fine." We started our songwriting experience as I asked Kara if there were things she would like to change about her life. She talked about being "normal" and a "regular kid." She spoke about missing being able to eat and drink (as her disease process had prevented her from eating by mouth for years at a time, and she was currently being fed via feeding tubes). In this experience, she was provided with a safe space to talk about things in her life that she would like to change.

I listened and jotted down ideas that she said, and we began to brainstorm on how to incorporate these thoughts into lyrics. "You see I would change my life . . ." This is how we started talking about ideas of things that she would like to change: "I wanna eat real food with the rest of my friends, and I wanna have candy too"; "I wanna go home and chill in my own house, don't wanna be told what to do"; "I don't wanna be on these meds no more, wanna walk without this pole [she points to the IV pole where she runs at least 10 different medication and nutrition infusions] . . ." "See these are the things I'd change, but I am still fine, fine, fine, fine, fine, fine . . ." [She repeated the original chorus right after.] We discussed knowing that some of these things could not change right now, but we also tried to keep the focus on some things that we could work on improving. Kara was happy to "freestyle" her new lyrics as I slowed down the groove and tapped out the beat on the back of my guitar. Her favorite line in the song became: "Keep your head up high/In yourself, believe in you, believe in me."

I counted on Kara's inspiration to write her own lyrics—or to substitute her own words into songs that she loves. We did lyric substitution experiences with India Arie's "Video," which contains the lyrics, "I'm not the average girl from your video and I ain't built like a supermodel, but I learned to love myself unconditionally because I am a queen." We also used the song "Control" by Janet Jackson, which says, "This is a story about control, my control. Control of what I say, control of what I do. And this time I'm gonna do it my way. 'Cause it's all about control. And I've got lots." We discussed what control meant to Kara and how we could come up with plans and effective ways to assert control over her medical condition, hospitalization, and life. Kara often played "Control" on days that she was feeling frustrated or upset. Sometimes she was upset about her condition, about pain, about her family, and at times it was more about being upset over the "normal" teenage things, such as a lights-out time, or restrictions on computers and video games. She substituted her own thoughts of control or restriction and belted it out to the groove we drummed out on hand drums.

Musical Improvisation

In improvisational experiences, the participants make up music spontaneously on the spot. Again, this process can involve singing or playing (using musical instruments, body parts, technology, or materials in the environment), and it may be very simple or quite complex musically and structurally. Improvisation can be created by an individual, a pair, or in a group. Improvisational experiences help to develop spontaneity and freedom, to deal with the unexpected, to attend to the here and now, to express emotions, to develop cognitive, motor, and social skills, and more.

Case Study: Adolescent Group—Psychiatric Unit

During my work with a group of adolescents on the psychiatric unit, we were exploring healthy ways of expressing difficult emotions. As a group, we decided to explore feelings of anger through musical improvisation. We discussed how feelings of anger build to a climax and then dissipate, in much the way a storm does. A large variety of tuned and untuned percussion instruments were available in the center of the group for them to choose from. Each group member had one or more instruments on which to play. Having improvised together several times, we decided to let the improvisation grow organically, with no one person leading it. They worked together to build the music to a climax. The music was chaotic and frenzied, yet had a controlled quality to it. After a while, the group started to bring the intensity of the music down, as if the anger was beginning to dissipate. All of a sudden, it began to build again, this time with even greater intensity. As I looked around, some of the group members seemed uncomfortable and stopped playing, while others seemed to be very engaged in making music, with their whole bodies involved. The music began to wane again, but as the sounds reduced in intensity, part of the group began to build the intensity again. This happened several times before the music eventually died down and stopped.

In the discussion after the improvisation, some of the group members shared how uncomfortable this level of intensity was for them. The chaos and unpredictability of the sounds, and its relationship to the chaos and unpredictability of anger in their experiences, made them feel very ill at ease. Most of those feeling that way were females in the group. Some members of the group discussed that the intensity was not enough for them and that they did not feel that it captured their feelings of anger and so had kept increasing the intensity each time it was dying down. Most of those feeling that way were males in the group. It led to a deeper discussion about different tolerance levels for different types of emotional expression. They also discussed unhealthy ways in which they have expressed their anger in the past and how improvising music in this way felt like a great way to express their feelings in a more healthy way.

Case Study: Grant—Radiation Oncology

Grant was a 7-year-old boy diagnosed with a brain tumor, who was receiving daily radiation treatments when I met him. After his treatment, Grant and his mother would come to the music therapy room to play. I laid out drums, shakers, a small harp, and a piano for him to choose from. Initially, Grant seemed to be drawn to various drums, some large and some small. I pulled up a chair next to him and asked if I could play with him. Without making eye contact, he nodded yes and pointed to a large conga drum, which was similar to the drum he chose for himself. At first Grant played the drum aggressively with loud and fast hand motions. I mimicked some of the sounds that he created while adding a few new ones, which he was able to quickly pick up and play back to me. This led to a musical game of "Simon Says," as he put it, or call and response (echoing) between us. Grant was able to lead and follow during this activity, not only playing loud and fast, but also exploring softer and slower sounds.

After a while, Grant stood up and began to explore other instruments. He found a large rainstick, which he pulled over to the other percussion instruments. He described the sound as a "storm" and suggested that we build our own storm. I brought out small and large ocean drums (drums that have tiny ball bearings that swirl around inside them and can sound like waves) and a thunder tube (an instrument that creates a thunder-like sound as you shake it). We sat on the floor exploring the sounds, when Grant assigned the instruments to his mother and me. Then he stood up and "directed" the storm. We created a storm that sounded very loud and chaotic at times, as Grant would jump and play loudly on the drums, thunder tube, and even pound the low end of the piano. At other times, the music was very soft and subtle, as only the rain stick was left sounding and the highest keys of the piano.

Grant then placed his instruments on the ground and said that he liked storms, but sometimes he liked what happened after storms, which he described as "sunny days to play outside in." When I asked if he would like to choose instruments to play what a "sunny day" might feel like, he chose a few small triangles, finger cymbals, the small harp, and the upper keys on the piano. Grant sat down at the piano and began to play the upper notes in a playful manner, which mimicked a jumping or skipping sensation. He instructed his mother and me to choose instruments to play as well. As before, while he played, he instructed us how to play, as he created music depicting hopping, running, and spinning. Grant and his mother continued to come to the music therapy room after his treatments for numerous sessions. Our musical experiences often led to verbal discussions, which may have been brought up in the play, from medical issues, emotions, things he missed doing at home, things he hated about the hospital, and even things he liked at the hospital.

Areas and Levels of Practice

As discussed here, music therapy addresses a multitude of need areas, including physiological, sensory, physical, cognitive, social, emotional, behavioral, spiritual, and musical. Music therapists work with people of all ages, from birth to old age, with a wide range of needs and concerns. Furthermore, music therapists are trained in a wide variety of theoretical orientations, including those that fall within didactic, recreational, medical, psychotherapeutic, ecological, and healing traditions (Bruscia, 1998, p. 158).

Within each area of practice, music therapists work at varying levels of therapeutic intervention (Bruscia, 1998, p. 162). That is, depending on the level and type of training that a music therapist receives, and the context within which a music therapist works, therapeutic interventions may occur at an auxiliary level (in which music is used for nontherapeutic but related purposes), an augmentative level (in which music therapy enhances other treatment modalities), an intensive level (in which music therapy takes a central role in the client's treatment), or a primary level (in which music therapy has an indispensable or singular role in the client's treatment) (Bruscia, 1998, p. 163).

PRACTICAL TECHNIQUES FOR NONSPECIALISTS

This section describes five different music techniques that could be utilized by nonspecialists with children and adolescents: a music listening and relaxation activity, a music performance activity, a music and movement activity, a lyric composition activity, and a music improvisation activity. For each activity we provide the therapeutic rationale, a description including materials used, and applications.

Music and Relaxation

"Up Goes the Castle"(www.youtube.com/watch?v=o6lgismLjeg)

Therapeutic Rationale

Young children often have difficulty relaxing. They also have difficulty understanding that when you breathe in, your abdomen expands and when you breathe out, it contracts. "Up Goes the Castle" (a *Sesame Street* song) allows children to relax in a fun, nonthreatening manner, and provides the instructions in a story about a King and Queen. This activity works well for children between the ages of 3 and 7.

Description

The materials that you will need are a recording of "Up Goes the Castle" by Ernie on the CD entitled *Bert and Ernie's Greatest Hits* and a foam castle.

The therapist tells the child to lie down with his or her back on the mat or the bed and listen to the story that Ernie is telling in the song. Tell the child to follow what Ernie says to do. Show the child how his or her stomach rises and falls during breathing.

The lyrics tell of a king and a queen who live in a castle on top of your stomach and that as you breathe in and out, they live high on a mountain and low to the ground, respectively. The imagery helps children breathe correctly for relaxation purposes. The song continues by having the king and queen argue about where it is better to live, until the person whose stomach it is explains that they have to keep breathing in and out. At the end, they agree that living both on a mountain and down in a valley is just fine. Given the content of the lyrics, the experience is both fun and instructive.

Applications

Up Goes the Castle can be used with children in hospital settings, children who have anxiety disorders, children with conduct problems, and children with attention-deficit/hyperactivity disorder. It is a fun way to help a child relax and learn to use good breathing techniques.

It could also be used for children who need to increase lung capacity, such as children with cystic fibrosis, asthma, or those who are post surgery.

Music Performing

Rock Band, Guitar Hero (video game systems include Wii, PlayStation, and Xbox 360).

Therapeutic Rationale

The adolescent age group can often be challenging to initially engage while trying to establish a therapeutic relationship. Many adolescents have a connection to music and/or video games, which is a great way to establish trust. Engaging in games such as Rock Band, Guitar Hero, and DJ Hero allows for a fun and lighthearted connection to build a trusting relationship as the individuals spend more time together in a nonthreatening situation. These games can also be played with more individuals, which can create a group or family experience.

Description

The materials you will need include:

- Game system that will run video games like Rock Band (Rock Band 2, Rock Band 3) and Guitar Hero
- Screen to play on (TV, projector)
- System controllers (mostly sold with the games)
- System-compatible game
- Track Packs allow you to enhance your song library in the game to more genre-specific songs, such as Country, Metal, Classic Rock
- Band-specific games include Green Day, AC/DC, the Beatles (Rock Band and Guitar Hero have similar series of genre-specific and band-specific versions of the game. Guitar Hero also has DJ Hero, which allows the player to experience being a DJ and exposes the genres of rap, hip-hop, and pop music.)

The therapist can engage in the game with the individual or group. The therapist can empower the adolescent(s) to make choices in the games to allow for trust building, as well as letting the child take a leadership role or decision-making role (which is something that is often taken away from hospitalized children).

Applications

Rock Band, Guitar Hero, DJ Hero, and similar video games (or even Karaoke) can be used with a variety of age groups (with a focus more on adolescents) and with a variety of diagnoses. It can be used in a pediatric medical setting as a tool for establishing trust and building a therapeutic relationship by creating a nonthreatening environment in which the individuals can play and communicate. It can also be a way to spark a child's musical interest in eventually learning an actual musical instrument. After playing these games, patients have often said they would like to move on to learning the actual instrument. It may be that the game gives them more self-confidence initially, and then they feel more able to tackle the real thing. Engaging in playing these musical games also helps develop fine and gross motor skills via muscle movement, standing to play a whole song, coordinating two hands doing independent motions, and sometimes feet as well.

Music and Movement

Therapeutic Rationale

Hospitalized children are often in need of increased physical activity, which can sometimes assist in the recovery/healing process from chronic illness, surgery, trauma, and extended hospitalizations. Music and movement can be utilized with a variety of age groups, ranging from toddlers to late adolescents, and can be used in co-treatment teams in the hospital, including members from physical and occupational therapy departments. Using music can often change the dynamic of the task from work to something that feels more fun and engaging to the patient.

Description

The materials you will need include a variety of audio recordings (to cover various age groups) and an audio playback system (CD player, MP3 player, iPod, iPad, etc.).

Examples of music to use:

"The Carnival of the Animals" (*Le carnaval des animaux*) by Camille
    Saint-Saens

"The Chicken Dance" by Werner Thomas

"Y.M.C.A." by The Village People

"Cupid Shuffle" by Cupid

"Cha Cha Slide" by DJ Casper (also known as Willie Perry)

"Electric Slide" by Marcia Griffiths

The Carnival of the Animals

This recording contains 14 musical selections, each with a different
title of an animal or place: Introduction and Royal March of the Lion;
Hens and Cockerels; Wild Asses; Tortoises; The Elephant; Kangaroos;
Aquarium; Persons with Long Ears; The Cuckoo in the Depths of the
Woods; Aviary; Pianists; Fossils; The Swan; and Finale. The play therapist can empower the patient to choose a movement from the list, as well
as a physical movement that coincides with the music that was chosen.
For example, a patient may choose "Tortoise" or "Kangaroo" and may
want to think of how each animal moves (slowly and deliberately; hopping and fast). The child and play therapist can talk about the movements these animals make as they imitate these animals while listening
to the music. In the music, the tempos, instrumentation, and composition reflect generalized characteristics of these animals, which can
reinforce the patient's movements leading to a fun and playful activity.

Line Dancing, Group Dancing, Called Instructions, and Freestyle Dance Movement Pieces

In using some of the aforementioned songs, specialists can involve both
younger and older patients in movement to music. These songs often
have called instructions directly in the lyrics involving both upper and
lower body movements (which could easily be adapted for each patient's
specific needs).

Applications

Music can be used as a playful and nonthreatening tool to assist patients
in increased/enhanced physical activity. Music and movement can

be utilized with a variety of age groups both in the individual or group settings.

Lyric Composition

Therapeutic Rationale

Patients may find it challenging to express their thoughts and emotions openly in the hospital for fear of many things. They are vulnerable and not in a position of power compared to the health professionals in this setting. Children often fear telling doctors/medical team members, and sometimes even family members, their thoughts and fears (e.g., what they don't like). Using a technique sometimes called lyric substitution, song augmentation, or piggybacking, the chosen familiar songs can often provide patients with structure and a format to express their emotions more freely and in a nonthreatening manner.

Description

The materials you will need are writing utensils, paper, and a copy of the original song lyrics. Taking away words and creating a fill-in-the-blank format can feel less overwhelming than creating a song from the ground up. This structure can create a structure in which patients can safely express their emotions. This technique can be tailored to fit the given age of patients by choosing a song that matches the patient's chronological or developmental age.

Example of a children's song: "Wheels on the Bus"
Traditional lyrics include:

The wheels on the bus go round and round
Round and round, round and round
The wheels on the bus go round and round
All through the town.

To create a lyric substitution opportunity, we could take away these words:

The _____ on/(in) the _____ go _____,

_____,_____

The _____ on/(in) the _____ go _____

All through the _____.

You can create as many verses as patients would like for this song. You can suggest to patients that they can brainstorm ideas, which may include things in the hospital, things at home, their favorite places, least favorite places, sights, sounds, smells, and so on.

For example:

> The nurse in my room says, "Take your meds!
> Take your meds, Take your meds!"
> The nurse in my room says, "Take your meds!"
> All through the hospital.

Another example, which is not specific to a hospital:

> The children at the park go jump slide swing
> Jump slide swing, jump slide swing
> The children at the park go jump slide swing
> All around the park.

Or, for older children, you could substitute the words to the tune of Queen's "We Will Rock You." The following is an example:
Verse:

> Billie is a patient make a big noise
> On the 7th floor gonna be a firefighter some day
> He's got his Superman shirt
> and his dog Max
> He can't want to see his friends in class.

Chorus:

> I can't wait to go home soon, home soon.
> I can't wait to go home soon, home soon.

Applications

This activity can be used in an individual or group setting being tailored to the age of the patient. That is, you would choose age-appropriate songs for which to substitute lyrics. It can be used to work through feelings associated with a procedure or situation or alternatively to distract children from the stressors of what they are coping with.

Improvisation/Storytelling With the Use of Instruments

Therapeutic Rationale

The storytelling process can be an empowering experience for patients and can be enhanced by the use of instruments and body percussion. Utilizing storytelling allows the patient to take on/assign different roles to characters as well as change and manipulate settings. Cognitive, emotional, and social skills can be focused on, as well as setting goals to increase creativity, communication, and self-esteem. Some patients may be more willing to share information or emotions through stories, characters, and play than through simply talking.

Description

The materials you will need are a variety of handheld percussion instruments and a variety of short stories. The children or adolescents can create a soundtrack for the story. Different instruments may represent different characters in the story and different events in the story. For example, hitting a woodblock three times could represent someone knocking on a door.

Fairy tales can be good to use with young children. Alternately, children or adolescents may enjoy making up a story on the spot and creating the sounds themselves or creating a story and having the group make the sound effects. A good strategy is to brainstorm the sounds before telling the story.

Applications

This technique can be used in a wide variety of situations. In a hospital setting, it might be good to have stories that represent the situation that the child or adolescent is facing at the time or alternately as a fun distraction from the stressors associated with what they are going through.

CONCLUSION

Although the research shows that it is preferable for a qualified music therapist to utilize musical experiences with children and adolescents who are dealing with various medical, emotional, behavioral, and mental health concerns, nonspecialists can also effectively incorporate music into their practice. With carefully thought out music techniques such as the ones described in this chapter, play therapists can effectively meet the needs of the children with whom they are working. We suggest, when possible, collaborating with a music therapist for the greatest possible effect.

SPECIALIZED TRAINING AND RESOURCES

Training in Music Therapy

In the United States, music therapists must hold at minimum a Bachelor's degree in music therapy. More than 70 music therapy training programs have been approved by the American Music Therapy Association. Within the initial training, 1,200 hours of clinical training must be completed, including a supervised internship. The American Music Therapy Association has developed a list of Professional Competencies for entry-level music therapists. Graduate programs in music therapy prepare music therapists for advanced clinical practice and research.

After completion of the training, music therapists must pass the national board certification exam for music therapists, in order to obtain the credential MT-BC (Music Therapist–Board Certified). This credential is granted through the Certification Board for Music Therapists (CBMT).

Credentialing in Music Therapy

Music therapists with advanced training often also have licensure such as Licensed Creative Arts Therapist (LCAT), Licensed Mental Health Counselor (LMHC), or Licensed Practicing Counselor (LPC). Many also have specialized training in a particular method of music therapy, such as Nordoff-Robbins Music Therapy (NRMT), Analytical Music Therapy (AMT), Neurological Music Therapy (NMT), Hospice and

Palliative Care Music Therapist (HPMT), Neonatal Intensive Care Unit Music Therapist (NICU-MT), or Fellow of the Association for Music and Imagery (FAMI).

Annual Music Therapy Conference(s) and Trainings

> Annual National Conference of the American Music Therapy Association
>
> Annual Regional Conferences of the American Music Therapy Association (NER, MAR, SER, SWR, WR, GLR)

Relevant Websites for Music Therapy

> American Music Therapy Association
> www.musictherapy.org
> Certification Board for Music Therapists
> www.cbmt.org
> Voices: A World Forum for Music Therapy
> www.voices.no
> World Federation for Music Therapy
> www.wfmt.info/WFMT/Home.html
> International Association for Music and Medicine
> www.iammonline.com

Media Clips From the American Music Therapy Association Website

> *MesotheliomaHelp.net* (January 2013): Music Therapy Can Speed Recovery Time in Mesothelioma Patients Undergoing Surgery
>
> *St. Charles County Surburban Journal* (October 2012): Music Therapy Has Educational Beat
>
> *Boston's NPR News* (October 2012): Music Therapists Help Ease Treatment of Children with Severe Burns
>
> *NewMediaChill.com* (September 2012): Harmony That Heals: Music Therapy's Mark in Medicine
>
> *Elephant Journal.com* (August 21, 2012): Drum Circles Aren't Just for Hippies: Using Music To Help Children's Spirits—One Beat at a Time

Dana-Farber Cancer Institute: Music Therapy Helps My Son Through Cancer Treatment

Science Daily (May 22, 2012): New Musical Pacifier Helps Premature Babies Get Healthy

About.com (May 15, 2012): Music Therapy in Neurology

About.com (May 12, 2012): The Musical Mind: How the Brain Appreciates Music

KOCO.com Oklahoma City (May 9, 2012): Music Therapy Aided OKC Brain Injury Sufferer

NBC Nightly News (April 9, 2012): Sparking Memories Musically

CNN iReport (April 1, 2012): Music Therapy and Autism: Amy's Challenging but Joyful Journey

Huffington Post Blog (March 15, 2012): Music Therapy Intervention in Medical Settings

National Stroke Association (March 14, 2012): Music Therapy . . . Something Beautiful Out of Something Devastating

PBS Newshour (February 27, 2012): The Healing Power of Music

PBS Newshour blog: A New Look at Music Therapy

Sam Houston State University: Music Therapist Works to Give Children With Autism a Voice

ABC News Nightline: Gabby Giffords Finding Voice Through Music Therapy, available on YouTube in three parts: Part I, Part 2, Part 3

National Public Radio's Science Friday (December 16, 2011): Treating Stress, Speech Disorders With Music

Huffington Post blog (January 9, 2012): Music Therapy in Early Childhood Classrooms

WebMD: Alan Cumming Tunes Into Music Therapy

Huffington Post Blog (July 21, 2011): Music Therapy: Global Perspectives

Cleveland.com: Music Therapy Eases Patients' Pain, Helps on Road to Recovery

ABC News: Facing Rehab: Exhaustion, Rehabilitation and Love

KHOU News: Initial Stages of Rehab Keeping Giffords Busy

The Boston Globe: When Language Is Blocked, Music May Offer Detour

Parade Magazine: Healing Sick Kids Through Music

Psychology Today: Music Therapy & Dyslexia: There's Still Hope

Pittsburgh Parent Magazine: Music Therapy Meets Special Needs

Chicago Tribune: Music Therapy: Teachers Strike an Emotional Chord With Disabled Students

PBS: Musical Minds

PBS: How Music Can Reach the Silent Brain

SpeechPathology.com: Music Therapy and the Emergence of Spoken Language in Children With Autism

NJ.com: Using the Language of Music to Speak to Children With Autism

Science Daily: Music Therapy May Offer for People With Depression

Star Bulletin: How Music Brings Peace

Star Bulletin: Drumming Beats the Blues Away

National Public Radio: Author Explains Mysteries of Music and the Mind

Nevada Appeal: Advocates Drum Up Support for Music Therapy Program

Star Bulletin: Music Makes Good Medicine

USA Today: Music Provides 'Audio Analgesic' for Some . . .

CBS Sunday Morning: Music Healing

NBC News, WILX: Music Therapy

New York Public Radio, WNYC: Music Is Medicine for Kids With Asthma

National Public Radio: Music Therapy May Help Ease Pain

ABC Eyewitness News, WABC-DT: The Healing Power of Music

Time Magazine: Music and the Mind

National Public Radio: Music Therapy

Relevant Music Therapy Books

Aldridge, D. (1996). *Music therapy research and practice in medicine: From out of the silence.* London, England: Jessica Kingsley.

Baker, F., Wigram, T., & Ruud, E. (2005). *Songwriting: Methods, techniques and clinical applications for music therapy clinicians, educators and students.* London, England: Jessica Kingsley.

Berger, D. S. (2002). *Music therapy, sensory integration and the autistic child.* London, England: Jessica Kingsley.

Brunk, B. K. (2000). *Music therapy: Another path to learning and communication for children in the autism spectrum*. Arlington, TX: Future Horizons.

Bruscia, K. E. (1991). *Case studies in music therapy*. Gilsum, NH: Barcelona.

Cassity, M. D., & Cassity, J. E. (2006). *Multimodal psychiatric music therapy for adults, adolescents, and children: A clinical manual* (3rd ed.). London, England: Jessica Kingsley.

Crowe, B. J., & Colwell, C. (2007). *Music therapy for children, adolescents, and adults with mental disorders*. Silver Spring, MD: American Music Therapy Association.

Edwards, J. (2007). *Music: Promoting health and creating community in healthcare contexts*. Newcastle, UK: Cambridge Scholars.

Edwards, J. (2011). *Music therapy and parent infant bonding*. Oxford, UK: Oxford University Press.

Froehlich, M. A. R. (1996). *Music therapy with hospitalized children*. Cherry Hill, NJ: Jeffrey Books.

Gardstrom, S. (2007). *Music therapy improvisation for groups: Essential leadership competencies*. Gilsum, NH: Barcelona.

Gilbertson, S., & Aldridge, D. (2008). *Music therapy and traumatic brain injury: A light on a dark night*. London, England: Jessica Kingsley.

Goodman, K. D. (2007). *Music therapy groupwork with special needs children: The evolving process*. Springfield, IL: Charles C. Thomas.

Grocke, D., Wigram, T., & Dileo, C. (2007). *Receptive methods in music therapy: Techniques and clinical applications for music therapy clinicians, educators and students*. London, England: Jessica Kingsley.

Hadley, S. (2003). *Psychodynamic music therapy: Case studies*. Gilsum, NH: Barcelona.

Hadley, S., & Yancy, G. (2011). *Therapeutic uses of rap and hip-hop*. New York, NY: Routledge.

Hanson-Abromeit, D., & Colwell, C. (2008). *Medical music therapy for pediatrics in hospital settings: Using music to support medical interventions*. London, England: Jessica Kingsley.

Kern, P., & Humpel, M. (2012). *Early childhood music therapy and autism spectrum disorders: Developing potential in young children and their families*. London, England: Jessica Kingsley.

Loewy, J. V. (1997). *Music therapy & pediatric pain*. Cherry Hill, NJ: Jeffrey Books.

Lorenzato, K. (2005). *Filling a need while making some noise: A music therapist's guide to pediatrics*. London, England: Jessica Kingsley.

Massicot, J. (2012). *Functional piano for music therapists and music educators: An exploration of styles*. Gilsum, NH: Barcelona.

McFerran, K. (2010). *Adolescents, music and music therapy: Methods and techniques for clincians, educators and students.* London, England: Jessica Kingsley.

Meadows, A. N. (2011). *Developments in music therapy practice: Case study perspectives.* Gilsum, NH: Barcelona.

Oldfield, A. (2006). *Interactive music therapy in child and family psychiatry: Clinical practice, research and teaching.* London, England: Jessica Kingsley.

Robb, S. (2003). *Music therapy in pediatric healthcare: Research and evidence-based practice.* Silver Spring, MD: American Music Therapy Association.

Standley, J. M. (2003). *Music therapy with premature infants: Research and developmental interventions.* Silver Spring, MD: American Music Therapy Association.

Streeter, E. (2001). *Making music with the young child with special needs: A guide for parents.* London, England: Jessica Kingsley.

Tomlinson, J., Derrington, P., Oldfield, A., & Williams, F. (2011). *Music therapy in schools: Working with children of all ages in mainstream and special education.* London, England: Jessica Kingsley.

Wigram, T. (2004). *Improvisation: Methods and techniques for music therapy clinicians, educators, and students* [Book and CD]. London, England: Jessica Kingsley.

Wolfe, D. E., & Waldon, E. G. (2009). *Music therapy and pediatric medicine: A guide to skill development and clinical intervention.* Silver Spring, MD: American Music Therapy Association.

Podcasts

AMTA-Pro is a series of music therapy podcasts by music therapists for music therapists. It can be found at: www.musictherapy.org/members/amtapro_entry_page/

REFERENCES

Abrams, B. (2010). Evidence-based music therapy practice: An integral understanding. *Journal Music Therapy, 47*(4), 351–379.

American Music Therapy Association. (2013). *What is music therapy?* Retrieved from www.musictherapy.org/about/musictherapy/

Association for Play Therapy—United States. (2013). *Play therapy defined.* Retrieved from www.a4pt.org/ps.playtherapy.cfm?ID=1158

Bradt, J., & Dileo, C. (2009). Music for stress and anxiety reduction in coronary heart disease patients (review). *The Cochrane Library,* Issue 2.

Bradt, J., Dileo, C., Grocke, D., & Magill, L. (2011). Music interventions for improving psychological and physical outcomes in cancer patients (review). *The Cochrane Library*, Issue 8.

Bradt, J., Magee, W. L., Dileo, C., Wheeler, B. L., & McGilloway, E. (2010). Music therapy for acquired brain injury (review). *The Cochrane Library*, Issue 7.

Bruscia, K. E. (1998). *Defining music therapy* (2nd ed.). Gilsum, NH: Barcelona.

Ginsberg, K. R. (2007). The importance of play in promoting healthy child development and maintaining strong parent-child bonds. *Pediatrics*, *119*(1), 182–191. doi: 10.1542/peds.2006-2697

Gold, C., Voracek, M., & Wigram, T. (2004). Effects of music therapy for children and adolescents with psychopathology: A meta-analysis. *Journal of Child Psychology and Psychiatry, and Allied Disciplines, 45*(6), 1054–1063.

Kemple, K. M., Batey, J. J., & Hartle, L. C. (2004, July). Music play: Creating centers for musical play and exploration. *Young Children*, 30–37.

Klassen, J. A., Liang, Y., Tjosvold, L., Klassen, T. P., & Hartling, L. (2008). Music for pain and anxiety in children undergoing medical procedures: A systematic review of randomized controlled trials. *Ambulatory Pedicatrics*, 8, 117–128.

Maratos, A. S., Gold, C., Wang, X., & Crawford, M. J. (2008). Music therapy for depression (review). *The Cochrane Library*, Issue 1.

McFerran, K. (2010). *Adolescents, music and music therapy: Methods and techniques for clinicians, educators and students*. London, England: Jessica Kingsley.

Pelletier, C. L. (2004). The effect of music on decreasing arousal due to stress: A meta-analysis. *Journal of Music Therapy, 41*(3), 192–214.

Standley, J. M., & Whipple, J. (2003). Music therapy with pediatric patients: A meta-analysis. In S. Robb (Ed.), *Music therapy in pediatric healthcare: Research and evidence-based practice* (pp. 19–30). Silver Spring, MD: American Music Therapy Association.

Wheeler, B. L. (2005). *Music therapy research* (2nd ed.). Gilsum, NH: Barcelona.

The Therapeutic Uses of Photography in Play Therapy

ROBERT IRWIN WOLF

INTRODUCTION

This chapter presents an historical overview of the development of photo-therapy, with specific emphasis on the integration of digital technology, but the suggested directives outlined may also be applied in a more traditional, less technological and digitally structured manner. A description of current possibilities, including the use of the most current application of contemporary technology, must be tempered with the understanding that technology has been expanding at an unprecedented rate and that, while we may be able to use what is available today, we need to use our own creativity, curiosity, and desire for innovation—in other words, *our ability to play with new technology*—in order to remain current. Readers are encouraged to keep abreast of current advances in related technologies. It is easy to become overwhelmed or intimidated if we allow ourselves to fall too far behind. However, if we overcome our initial discomfort with change, we will be able to explore and *play* with new ways to integrate

Parts of this chapter have been reproduced, with permission, from "Advances in Phototherapy Training," by R. I. Wolf, 2007, *The Arts in Psychotherapy, 34* , pp. 124–133.

technologies that our clients, especially children and adolescents, have most likely already learned and utilize on a daily basis.

What I outline here today may well become obsolete next week. When this author first began writing about the use of Polaroid cameras in the art therapy process (Wolf, 1976, 1978, 1983), digital cameras, home color printers, smartphones with cameras, and portable digital tablets were not only unavailable, but *inconceivable* as innovative technologies that would later become totally integrated into our current life and transform the world as they have today. So what will be part of our technical life in five years? We cannot possibly know today. The best we can do is attempt to keep abreast of new things as they come along and be aware of other professionals in the field as they discover new ways of using the photographic modality in their therapeutic work (Weiser, 2010). We need only to do a Google search on "Photo Therapy" to find a rich resource of articles on this subject.

We also discuss the uses of other technologies, such as online blogs and other interactive posting and communication possibilities, that might enhance the group process within the play therapy experience. This chapter provides a listing of phototherapy techniques that can be used in play therapy, but we must always be aware that the technique must be thoughtfully modified to fit within the practitioner's theoretical framework. This chapter attempts to offer a preliminary opportunity to see how some techniques have been successfully applied to clinical work with case studies from graduate students' clinical work with child and adolescent clients that illustrate some possibilities of application. These directives must be understood as extremely powerful clinical techniques that must be used with caution, even though the overall environment that we create may initially seem playful. The practice of any form of psychotherapy requires intense clinical training, regardless of one's theoretical orientation. It is ultimately our ability to understand and process the communication coming from our clients that leads to the effectiveness of any therapeutic modality. I offer here a brief description of what I believe to be the theoretical foundation for the use of photographic images in an art/play therapy environment, but this is not meant to replace the foundation provided by other more extensive clinical training that is required before any technique may be successfully and ethically implemented into actual treatment.

HISTORICAL OVERVIEW

Phototherapy is a relatively new specialization within the field of art/play therapy and psychotherapy. Although its initial use was predominantly documentary in nature—psychiatrists would take photographs of mental patients before and after treatment—we have evolved and integrated photographic media within the structure of the psychotherapeutic treatment process, enabling clients to create powerful visual metaphors that are then used to achieve deeper self-understanding and personal insight *during the treatment process.* If we encourage our clients to play with these metaphors, then we have established a safe way for them to externalize conflicts and manipulate them in a way that promotes mastery of unconscious conflict without having to directly face their issues in a way that would trigger defenses and, in some cases, a nonproductive regression.

Another way to see this is that we promote an acting in, within the artwork, rather than an acting out, a behavior that is often seen in adolescence when a feeling is converted into an action and becomes less available and more difficult to confront and process in a productive way (Rexford, 1978). Because this chapter demonstrates only a few ways to process phototherapy directives, it is important to be aware that many of the exercises described here may also be modified for use within a variety of other theoretical orientations. As examples we might consider the differences and similarities between *Play Therapy*, as described by Virginia Axline (1947), *Art as Therapy*, as described by Edith Kramer (1971), and *Play as Therapy*, as described by D. W. Winnicott (1971).

Axline (1947) and Kramer (1971) both describe a form of treatment that was basically nondirective, relying on the natural tendency of children to use play as a way to express and work through emotional issues that were creating anxiety. The postulate was that if you create a safe space, whatever needs to come out will emerge, and children's innate ability to resolve their own issues through play and expressive artwork would prevail. Winnicott (1971) took this idea and developed it further within the psychoanalytic framework, opening the door to a theoretical foundation for art and expressive therapies. His seminal work, *Playing and Reality* (Winnicott, 1971), posits a similar notion that play, as a natural innate function that is easily seen in children, is often lost as one grows older and undergoes the influence of society's pressures toward developing more cognitively, less creatively, and disregarding one's own deeper levels of unconscious experience. This was an expansion on the earlier Freudian theories that focused mostly on the damaging consequence of disconnection from the unconscious and the need to bring unconscious conflict into consciousness.

As a pediatrician and psychoanalyst, Winnicott was well versed in Freudian theory. By observing mothers and children in his pediatric practice, he was able to add his own unique contribution to the earlier idea that unconscious conflict always seeks expression (Freud, 1943), with his emphasis on the importance of play and creativity as a vehicle for improving mental health (Winnicott, 1968). He went further to state that therapy required the reteaching of our clients how to play and went on to describe a theoretical foundation for his observations that include the concept of transitional objects, transitional space as the precursor to play, and description of the qualities of "good-enough mothering" (Winnicott, 1960) that lead to the establishment of this creative space. He postulated from a psychoanalytic perspective that this original creative space is what we, as psychoanalytic therapists, attempt to recreate as a prerequisite for any effective therapeutic treatment.

So we can see that while there may be two distinct directions in the way we may apply these techniques, the use of creativity has emerged within our respective professional fields as the foundation for the application of creative process in achieving mental health through this common conceptual origin: *the value of play.* We understand that by offering our clients the use of play to identify and exercise mastery of unconscious conflict, they may eventually repair emotional damage through the expression of creative visual metaphors, perhaps at times simply by this expressive quality without insight, or in more psychoanalytic treatment, with insight.

PHOTOGRAPHY AS A THERAPEUTIC MODALITY: THE POWER OF THE IMAGE

Our first experience of the world around us is filtered though our sensory apparatus: visual, olfactory, tactile, and auditory. We concern ourselves here with our visual perception. For the young child, visual images may not at first be understood, but they may become connected with strong affect. Later in life, all types of visual images may speak to us on this primal level of communication and often generate strong affective reactions that may circumvent secondary process defenses. The photographic image often offers less resistance than other forms of art expression for use as a therapeutic modality, especially in adolescents, because it circumvents resistance that stems from a developmental tendency toward perfectionism and its concomitant fear of failure. Adolescents are more likely to be comfortable picking up a camera and taking photographs than they are facing an empty canvas. This is an unfortunate consequence of both societal/peer pressure (external forces) and developmental phenomena (internal forces).

Adolescents experience this shift from drawing internalized images to attempting to observe and reproduce their outer world through drawing—the shift from intellectual realism to visual realism (DiLeo, 1983; Luquet, 1913) or preconceptual to concrete operational (Piaget, 1954). This often leads adolescents to give up more traditional art materials as they pass through this developmental phase and become frustrated with their sudden awareness of the disparity between what they see outside and what they create in their art. If we offer photography to adolescents, they may find it more easily used than traditional art materials to externalize their deeper conflicts through visual metaphors that they inevitably create.

THE IMPORTANCE OF THE UNCONSCIOUS

Our unconscious is constantly picking up, absorbing, and processing information from the world around us. Some of our day-to-day experiences may create some tension within us, and this tension is converted into anxiety, which then seeks some form of expression. The ego resists direct expression of conflict and relies on other more indirect methods of expression, such as manifesting psychological symptoms, slips of the tongue, or dreams (Freud, 1913). To this I would add that the creation of a safe space and the introduction of art or, in our case, photographic materials also provides a transitional space (Winnicott, 1975) within which whatever is seeking expression will emerge through a visual metaphor. It is interesting that our study of how dreams convert unconscious conflict into visual images—through condensation, displacement, symbolization, and so on (Freud, 1913)—may also serve as a guide for us to understand visual images that occur in artwork, including photographs.

THE RANGE OF PROCESSING VISUAL METAPHORS

Although we may decide that it is best for our clients that we remain simply a witness to their creative expression of their unconscious material as it emerges from an effective phototherapy intervention, our intervention may be required sometimes. The key to effective therapeutic intervention always lies in the hands of the clinician. In the case of processing photographic material, this may, in addition to the extensive clinical training referred to earlier, require the skill of the clinician to integrate the technology into the theoretical orientation that is determined by prior clinical training. A Gestalt therapist would certainly work differently from a Freudian psychoanalyst or an expressive art therapist. One's own ability to process within a particular modality may be determined by the degree of comfort the clinician has with that particular modality. A higher degree of comfort may be achieved *by the clinician* by first exploring the modality, before attempting its use with clients.

A NOTE OF CAUTION

The directives outlined as follows must first be fully integrated into the clinician's theoretical focus for them to be effectively utilized. As stated previously, these seemingly playful exercises, under the proper circumstances, elicit powerful unconscious material. These techniques are designed to circumvent secondary process defense mechanisms and tap directly into primary process material. This material may be guarded by mechanisms that create safe visual metaphors. The clinician must determine if the client would then benefit from further understanding of the symbolic meaning of this material, or if the client's ego would become overwhelmed by such an effort. Good therapy always carefully considers this question. We must be careful as clinicians, who are often quite eager to demonstrate the power of our techniques and the effectiveness of our clinical skill, to remain focused on our client's ability to constructively utilize what we offer and not inadvertently act out our own personal needs. We must respect defense mechanisms as we attempt to replace rigidly restrictive ones with higher level defenses that are more flexible, enabling the achievement of a healthier, more adaptable ego structure (Freud, 1967).

So I caution the reader to respect the power of these directives and their ability to quickly create a window into your client's deepest unconscious world, which may be filled with fantasies and conflict. Your challenge will be to demonstrate your ability to simply listen, hear, understand, and ultimately respond in a way that is most helpful to your client. These exercises may also be used simply as playful activities without any intervention by the therapist, but we must always be aware of their deeper potential power. Our astute clinical judgment, made out of this respect for the power of this modality and an assessment of our client's level of ego functioning, should inform our decision about how to work with what our client produces. From a psychoanalytic perspective, we would only intervene when we sense a resistance, and then encourage our client to process and understand what lies behind it. Our clients are often able to work on their own material if we simply create a safe space within which they can allow whatever needs to emerge, to present itself. This space requires clear boundaries, which are often achieved only after a series of testing is responded to without retaliation but with the consistent reiteration of consequences for their actions and the demonstration of the therapist's ability to follow through, the maintenance of consistency of time and space, the establishment of rules (for groups), and the demonstration of your ability to listen with genuine curiosity and nonjudgmental interest.

For higher functioning children and adolescents, we may consider offering the opportunity to explore creative digital phototherapy projects by providing the technical support necessary to develop proficiency in digital editing. Here we can demonstrate to clients how these techniques work and provide *visceral* experiences that inform them of the power of this modality on an *affective* as well as cognitive level (Wolf, 1990). An important potential goal of an art/play phototherapy experience should involve the development of creativity and not focus just on pathology. This approach is consistent with the concept of self-actualization, as described by the Human Potential Movement spearheaded by writers/ clinicians such as Maslow in the 1960s (Maslow, 1967) and ego psychologists such as the Blanks in the 1980s (Blank & Blank, 1979). *Sublimation*, which is what we are trained to help develop in our clients, is seen by ego psychologists as the highest level of ego defense mechanisms and, as such, is the least restrictive (Freud, 1967). As play/ phototherapists, we have a unique opportunity to help these clients focus on enhancing their emotional health through introspection and insight by helping to develop their creativity.

TECHNOLOGICAL UPDATE

As stated previously, the very best anyone can do today is to give you an overview of what already exists and encourage you to continue to explore possibilities for the discovery of new potential uses of technology. New possibilities are available every day, and it is up to us to remain well-informed. For example, if we type *Photo Apps for Smart Phones* into a Google search, we receive a seemingly endless numbers of choices. Each of these apps could be explored and their therapeutic implication discovered. Today, many of our child and adolescent clients rely heavily on this type of technology to feel literally connected to their social world. The use of social networks, e-mail, Twitter, and others too numerous to identify here have become a way of life for our younger generations. To find a way to integrate these technologies into our phototherapy treatment will remain a constant challenge for us as the options continue to expand daily. So let me outline a few possibilities with the understanding that these are just the beginning.

Many digital editing apps are either free or very inexpensive and can be downloaded directly to your smartphone or digital tablet. Some that immediately come to mind are Snapseed (for instant access to quick, basic creative editing functions from your smartphone) and Instagram (for instant sharing of photographs as they are taken). You need to be aware that there will be different versions for each platform, which are at this time either Apple or Android operating systems. Some apps are available for only one platform or the other, so be aware of this limitation if you are working within a group. You would need to make sure that it would be available for all members before suggesting it.

There are online digital editing programs like photo online sharing communities, such as Flikr, Google Picasa Web Albums, or Shutterfly, for posting of photographs that could be used by clients to present their work online during the time between sessions. This may be particularly interesting for group projects. You may want to consider setting up a Yahoo! chat group, an online blog using free open-source software such as Blogger or Wordpress, or a similar online forum, where members could post their images and comment on each other's work online. Technical support and other types of feedback can also be provided by you or other group members through this mechanism. Participants should be encouraged to offer their feedback to each other's postings in the format of user comments, such as "If this were my image, it would mean . . . to me," similar to the method of processing dream material proposed by Montegue Ullman. This technique provides a structure where clients can receive supportive feedback in a nonintrusive manner and promotes optimal use of the online format (Ullman & Zimmerman, 1987).

When using cameras in smartphones, tablets, or actual digital cameras, images can then be attached to e-mails and sent to desktop computers for more elaborate editing that these smaller devices might not be capable of. This transfer to computer would also enable clients to introduce many other creative editing effects, like adding text to an image or applying various filters, that might be required for some of the projects listed later. You may want to set up a secured, password-protected wireless network in your treatment space that enables clients to wirelessly send photographic images to a wireless printer, or to a larger computer first for greater editing possibilities. Small printers provide a docking mechanism that allows one to simply connect a smartphone directly and print a four-by-six-inch photo (but without much editing capability).

There are many new resources for learning more about the technological adaptations of photography in psychotherapy that may be of interest. Two particularly valuable ones are a Facebook group on Therapeutic Photography (https://www.facebook.com/groups/PhotoTherapy.and.Therapeutic .Photography) and a website: www.Phototherapy-Centre.com

SPECIAL CONSIDERATIONS
OF CONFIDENTIALITY

When working with clients in any clinical setting, considerations of confidentiality must always be maintained. If you are working without an online component, appropriate release forms must first be considered as an essential part of the initial requirements for your treatment when using this modality. In addition, if you are working *with* an online component, further considerations must be made. In some cases, clear limitations on what types of images may be posted online may be needed. For example, you may want to carefully select only options that do not require photos that expose the specific identity of clients. You may also need to set other restrictions on the content or nature of any photos posted online. The online component must be used in conjunction with your *in-person group* sessions, where clients have an opportunity to present their projects in a hard-copy form and receive face-to-face interactive feedback from the other group participants. The online experience gives participants an opportunity to warm up for the more intimate face-to-face group experiences. Group sessions can be profoundly powerful experiences for all participants.

It is interesting to consider how the following exercises may be modified for application with different client populations. The instructions might be simplified or elaborated for specific clients or groups, but the actual processing would require the therapist to first evaluate a client's ego functioning in order to create an appropriate therapeutic environment that is uniquely suited for their client. The client's capacity for insight, introspection, and self-awareness would determine the extent and depth of this processing. Some clients would benefit from simply an ego-supportive experience, whereas others might benefit from a more in-depth approach.

Other variables also need to be taken into account when planning to implement any of the following directives for use with digital photographic technology with specific clients. First, their technical skill or ability to learn technical processes must be assessed. As this may vary among clients, great care should be taken to not overwhelm or frustrate clients. Potential for acting out must also be assessed and precautions taken to prevent damage to equipment or other clients. Also, availability and access to equipment may influence the actual structure of these experiences. For example, if you are planning to work in a group format and the number of cameras, computer terminals, and printers is limited, then the structure of these activities must be modified for practical reasons. The therapist may then need to take the photographs, print them out in hard copy, and have a group use traditional art materials to modify and elaborate the images. In these instances, the spontaneity of the digital technology for simply taking and quickly printing, rather than the creative use of editing software, would be the main advantage over more traditional film photography.

Having more highly functioning clients process these exercises once they are finished provides them with a powerfully significant affective experience that will enable them to understand, on a visceral level, what they are unconsciously struggling with.

SUGGESTIONS FOR CREATIVE PROJECT DIRECTIVES

The following list of possible projects may be offered to your clients to choose from. Although many are listed here in a digital format, they may all be modified to reduce their technological dependence based on the access to equipment or to accommodate more specific client needs. Any directives may be completed either with digital equipment and editing software or with hard-copy photos and basic art materials. The Adobe Photoshop professional software package (currently CS6), although expensive, offers a wide variety of functions that produce effects that are similar to a variety of art materials. The Adobe *Photoshop Elements* program is available at a more reasonable cost and has many of the functions that are likely to be needed by your clients. Photographs may be taken by the client or found on open-source photo sites such as Google Images, where a huge variety of images, selected by category, may be found and downloaded for use within these projects.

For more advanced and sophisticated clients, you can find online a variety of self-publishing websites, such as Blurb.com, Lulu.com, and Createspace.com. These publishers offer free software that can be

downloaded onto your computer. They provide a template for upload-
ing your images and text into a format that may then be used to print a
book. These sites usually offer many different options for size, page limit,
and price and usually allow you to initially print just one book. The
template can be left online for future purchases by the author or other
friends, relatives, or interested parties. The results can be quite impressive. One final note: When you are using original photo files for creative
projects, it is important to remember that when you are finished with
your elaboration, you should always press "SAVE AS" and never "SAVE"
because pressing the "SAVE" button will erase your original file by copy-
ing over it with your modified project.

Here are some suggestions for Projects:

(Readers should be advised that the following directives are taken
from Adobe Photoshop software. Users can employ other variations of
these techniques from other available non-Adobe software.)

1. *Self-portraits*: Create a photographic portrait of yourself, leaving
space for a large white background area. Using digital elaboration, write
or draw a reaction to what you see, directly on the photo. *This can be
accomplished in Photoshop by selecting one of the Lasso or Pen tools and out-
lining the subjects. Then, using the Move tool, place the subject on a new,
white background. The Paintbrush tool may then be used to paint or draw on
the image by selecting different effects that mimic paint, chalk, or line, and the
T text tool may be used to add text to the image.*

2. *Collages*: Use digital editing functions to create collages that
express visual metaphors or express a particular feeling. *You may wish
to combine these photos with other art media. You may use the functions
described above to cut out images from their original background and move
them to other images. Once you begin building layers, you may play with the
opacity tool and various filters to create various effects with each layer.*

3. *Creative dyad*: Pick a partner, and set up and photograph a pose
where you are both interacting. Elaborate in a way that communicates
or emphasizes some aspect of this relationship. Add cartoon captions to
express an imaginary dialogue. *Use the tools from item #1 to place both subjects on a white background. Select the size and placement of each person by
using the Transform tool (keyboard shortcuts: Ctrl-T on Windows, Cmd-T*

on Mac). Then use other photos or digital paintbrush to add a new background. Use the T type tool (keyboard shortcut: T on Windows and Mac) to add dialogue. Draw cartoon captions around the words with a small brush tool.

4. *Monster-self*: Create yourself as a monster. *Start with a photo of yourself and use a variety of filters to change and distort yourself into a monster.*

5. *True-self, false-self portrait*: Create a pair of photographs, one that represents aspects of your "true self" (the one you feel you really are) and one that represents your "false self" (the one you show to others but does not feel authentic). *Use a variety of functions from the Filter menu along with the Liquify filter to make changes to the original photos of yourself.*

6. *Self-image construct*: Create a photographic construct that symbolically represents you without using a direct image of yourself. *Use a variety of your own or open-source photographs and digital editing functions to create your image. Laminate photos to a rigid material like foam core or illustration board and build a three-dimensional construction with these images.*

7. *Creative portrait poster*: Create a full-size photograph of yourself holding a blank paper in front of your body. Once the photo is printed, draw in the blank space indicating how you see yourself or how you would like your body to look. *Use the Paintbrush tool to draw within the white space, or add other images using your Move tool.*

8. *Favorite pet*: Take a photo of an animal that you would like to have as a pet. *Use digital software to elaborate and change this animal so it would be able to be your pet.*

9. *Superhero*: Create a Superhero starting with a photograph of yourself. *Use creative digital editing functions to create a superhero. Use the Type function tool to describe your superpowers.*

10. *Inside/outside self-constructs*: Using photographs mounted to cardboard or foam core, create a boxlike structure that reflects how you experience your inner self and also how you present yourself to the outside world, in one combined form. *This is similar to the True-self/False-self project, with the addition of adding the images to a three-dimensional structure.*

11. *Wanted poster*: Take a front and side-view photo of yourself or someone you know and make a Wanted Poster from those mug shots. Then, below the image, describe the crime that this outlaw is guilty of committing. *Use the Lasso or Pen tools and the Move tool to place your*

photo on a new background. This may be the scene of the crime or a plain white background. Use the T type tool to write out a description of your crime, along with the Reward!

12. *Creative mobile constructions*: Create three-dimensional constructs using images printed on paper and then laminated to cardboard or foam core. Explore various methods of construction and design some method to exhibit your constructs. Design a way that they can be made into a mobile and hung from the ceiling.

13. *Creative story*: Tell something that you have never before been able to tell about yourself through photography. This may be done in one photographic image or several, in a storyboard format. *Use the Move tool to place different figures on a new background. Add additional elements to complete your story.*

14. *Photobook*: Using a sequence of photographs and digital art media, create a book that tells a significant story about yourself. *Elaborate on the Creative Story project by adding additional pages to your story. With more advanced adolescents, you may be able to use a self-publishing website to upload images and text to their platform and have an actual book printed.*

15. *Creative home*: Photograph your current or childhood home. Laminate photographs of the exterior and interior to cardboard or foam core and make a miniature reconstruction. Creatively elaborate in a way that changes the environment. *Use the tools from the Creative Construct directive and then resize your wall using the Image drop-down menu to find Image Size function, so each wall section will properly fit together. Add elements to the original photo of each section with your editing software before laminating the sections to construction material.*

16. *Group/family portrait*: Photograph your family or group. Develop some creative way to have members react to themselves and/or other family members. *Use the functions above in the Creative Dialogue directive to have people speak to each other. Use the Lasso tool to remove people and the Move tool to move them around or add new people.*

17. *Transparency elaboration*: Print an image on a piece of transparent photographic media and creatively explore the material. *Use a variety of filters to explore this effect.*

18. *Image transfer to clothing*: Create an image that you want to transfer to an article of clothing. Flip your image 180 degrees horizontally in Photoshop and then print it onto a special photographic transfer

material. Carefully follow directions from an online tutorial or supplied printing manual and use an iron to complete the transfer onto fabric.

19. *Childhood snapshot reconstructions*: Re-photograph using a digital camera or digitally scan a series of childhood snapshots and then, using creative techniques, reconstruct the photos in a new way. *Use a combination of digital editing techniques and visual art materials.*

20. *Secret story*: Take a photo of someone who you want to tell something that you never told them before and tell them the story through pictures. *Use the Lasso and/or Pen tools and the Move tool to cut out the person from their background and set him or her in a new place. Then add images that tell your story. You can add words with the T type tool.*

21. *Mask/costume image*: Start with a photo of yourself. *Use the Paintbrush tool to paint over the figure and add a mask and/or a costume to cover yourself.*

22. *Inanimate/animate object*: Take a photo of an inanimate object and make it into an animate object. *Use the Paintbrush tool to add things like facial features, arms, and legs to your inanimate object.*

23. *New room*: Take a photo of your room and make it change into what you would like it to be in five years. *Use Filters, Paintbrush tools, or add other images to create the desired effect.*

24. Take a photo of something that you:

Fear
Hate
Love
Wish you had
Wish you didn't have

Use a variety of editing functions to elaborate on this image in some way.

DETAILED DIGITAL EDITING DIRECTIONS FOR MORE ADVANCED PROJECTS

The following are just a few more detailed examples of how digital media and editing processes may be utilized to create these exercises. Clients may be simultaneously taught how to use more elaborate digital editing software while exploring projects that are designed to elicit unconscious material.

25. *Body language exploration:* Choose a full-body image of yourself. Remove the figure from the background. Place the image onto a new white background. Take a few moments to carefully look at the image. Imagine that this figure is *not* you. Examine the body language and let your imagination find a new place and activity for "this person." Elaborate on where this person is and what he or she is doing.

   a. File> Open> select a photo with a clearly defined figure as a subject > OK

   b. Image> Image size: Set size to 72 dpi × 8.5″ × 11″ > OK

   c. File> New (to create a blank new canvas). Set size to 72 dpi × 8.5″ × 11″ > OK

   d. Click on your subject image and then click the Magnetic Lasso icon and carefully outline the subject, clicking every 1/16th of an inch as you go. Return to the starting point and click.

   e. When you get a vibrating dotted line around your subject, click Edit> Copy. Click on your blank canvas, and then click Edit> Paste.

   f. Use the Move tool to relocate the image onto the new blank canvas.

   g. Use the keyboard shortcuts (Ctrl-T on Windows, Cmd-T on Mac) for the Transform function tool to resize and move your subject.

   (Note: Freely Transforming an object in Photoshop results in the following for layers: Scaling, Rotating, Skewing, Distorting, etc. These advanced functions may require online tutorials for better understanding.)

   h. Use the Paintbrush tool (keyboard shortcut, B on Windows/Mac) to draw in a new background in the blank space left around the original image.

   i. Use the Liquify filter to add any desired distortion to the figure.

26. *Autobiographical Book Cover/CD cover design:* Select a photograph of yourself and use it in a design for either a cover for an autobiography of your life or a CD of music that you have written and/or recorded.

    a. All of the tools in previous exercises plus the Type tool (Keyboard shortcut, T on Windows/Mac from the left sidebar) for adding text to your image

    b. Go to Filter drop-down menu and explore the various creative functions to create artistic effects.

    c. Go to Image drop-down menu and click on the Adjustments submenu to find another large drop-down menu. Explore the various functions available there, especially the Levels, Posterize, and Curves functions.

27. *First memory or dream photo construction:*

    a. Open a photo to be used as a background for this image. Adjust the image size to 72 dpi × 8.5″ × 11″.

    b. Open other photos that you wish to add to the original background. Use the Magnetic Lasso or Magic Wand tools to select parts from the secondary photos that you wish to add to the background. Use the Move tool to relocate these images. Use the keyboard shortcuts (Ctrl-T on Windows, Cmd-T on Mac) to freely transform the image to the correct size and position.

    c. Use the Opacity function from each layer to adjust the visibility of each.

    d. Use the paintbrush tool to elaborate.

    e. Flatten layers.

    f. Use the Smudge tool to blend forms together.

    The following are some simple projects that may be used while completely avoiding the use of any photographic material containing an image of your client.

28. Take a photo of a place and write a story about what it would be like to be there.

29. Take a photo from a magazine and add something to it.

30. Take a photo of a person and make up a story about him or her.

CASE STUDIES: CLINICAL AND CREATIVE USES OF PHOTOGRAPHY

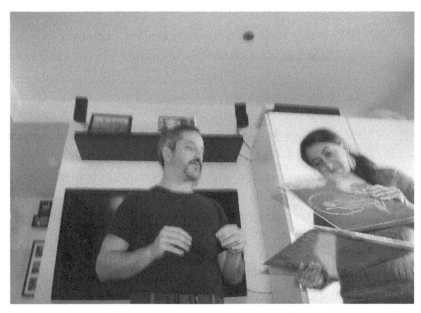

Figure 8.1   Candid photo by 3-year-old

Expanding the Definition of Mental Health: Promoting Emotional Growth, Not Only Curing Illness

I'd like to take this opportunity to offer another valuable application of photography as a way to *enhance the natural process* of child development, in addition to the clinical uses that would be focused more on *correcting problems* that may occur within this process. All too often today, we in the mental health field have aligned ourselves with the medical treatment model that focuses on identifying and curing illness. We have lost our roots in the human potential movement, which originally emphasized the growth-producing effect of creativity in normal human development.

The role of empathy in healthy parenting has been shown to facilitate emotional growth (Grolnick, 1990; Kohut & Wolf, 1978; Miller, 1981). In this brief case study (see Figure 8.1), the author gave a camera to his 3-year-old grandson at a family get-together, who then spontaneously took this candid photograph of his father and aunt. This seemingly innocent image, which was not posed, allowed his parents, as well as his extended family, to become more sensitized to how he perceives the world around him. This promoted empathy and will greatly enhance their appreciation of the challenges this small child faces as he navigates within a world that is typically designed for much larger people.

Graduate Students' Case Study

The Directive: *"Take an Image of Yourself, Place It on a Different Background, and Reflect on Its Meaning"*

"I chose to create multiple images of my face growing from a tree, looking down at one of my faces falling from the tree (Figure 8.2). As I reflected on the image I thought of apples ripening and falling from the branches of a tree. When they are ready and ripe, they will fall on their own. I related the image and associations to my current stage in life as a graduate student. It was the beginning of my final semester of college. I was near the point of graduation and was nearly finished with my studies and internship. I was ripening and becoming ready to fall from the tree, which was symbolic of the nurturance I received

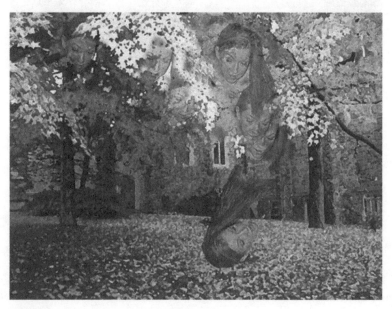

Figure 8.2   Image of Self

from my classes and supervisors. I was becoming ready to provide nurturance to the clients who I will eventually work with. It also symbolized loss, as I was working on detaching myself from unhealthy personal relationships."

The Directive: *"Create a Self-Portrait Using Digital Editing and Reflect on Its Meaning"*

"The face was white and surrounded by black. I took the photograph when I was depressed, and I hated the way I felt. I felt self-pity, self-doubt, self-hatred, pessimistic, trapped, angry, and lethargic. Depression has always been in and out of my life and my ideal self is able to fight it off, work through it, and have hope. My 'bad self' is trapped inside of it; unmoving. I presented the collages to my classmates, and I became emotional for the first time toward one of my phototherapy pieces. The images on the 'bad self' collage had to do with patterns of abuse that

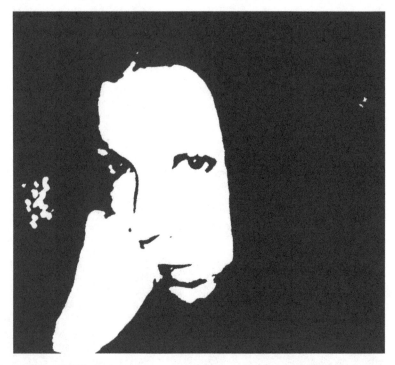

Figure 8.3   Self-Portrait

have been handed down, generation to generation, in my family. My grandmother was physically and emotionally abused, as was my mother, as were my sisters, and as I was, when I had, in the past, chosen to involve myself in abusive relationships. I never want to go back to that place and I never want to repeat that pattern. I spoke about my sister and her addiction, my mother's co-dependency, my father's abuse toward her, and my survivor's guilt. The class was extremely supportive and offered compassionate feedback, which helped me to see that it was okay for me to not make the same decisions that they made and continue to choose to make."

CONCLUSION

Phototherapy has been around in one form or another since the advent of the camera. It has only recently, with the wider use and lower prices of computers and digital editing equipment, taken on more universal interest within the play/art therapy community as a viable new modality. In the past, the implementation of phototherapy within a therapeutic environment required the physical establishment of a photographic darkroom, and art/play therapists typically did not have the resources available to implement this type of film-based phototherapy component into their practice.

The illustrative case studies described in this chapter have demonstrated how digital and hard-copy photographic media may be integrated into play therapy treatment. Although the examples and illustrations offered here reflect only a very small sample population, all of the exercises offered may be modified for use with various client populations in a variety of clinical settings.

SPECIALIZED TRAINING AND RESOURCES

There is no specific certifying body or organization for the field of Phototherapy. Judy Weiser's Phototherapy Centre (www.Phototherapy-Centre.com) offers training seminars, workshops, and courses through

Southwestern College, which lead to a certificate through that organization. The College of New Rochelle, where Bob Wolfe (author of this chapter) is a professor in the graduate Art Therapy Master's degree program, also offers a certificate in Phototherapy for students who minor and specialize in Phototherapy as part of their Master's degree training.

As for video resources, "Phototherapy Techniques" is available through Phototherapy Centre (Phototherapy-Centre.com). The websites for the central professional organizations and conferences readers could join or attend to become a part of this field and receive professional development are www.Photovoice.org and International PhotoTherapy Association online databases at www.uia.be/s/or/en/1100040085 For central books/ journal articles/monographs that readers are recommended to find on Phototherapy, please visit the Phototherapy Centre Website (www .Phototherapy-Centre.com).

The ethics guidelines for this field are similar to those of Art Therapy, with the additional caution that careful thought should be given to the confidentiality of client artwork generated through phototherapy, because the identities of clients and their subjects may be compromised by the photographic element.

REFERENCES

Axline, V. M. (1947). *Play therapy*. New York, NY: Ballantine Books.

Blank, G., & Blank, R. (1979). *Ego psychology I*. New York, NY: Columbia University Press.

DiLeo, J. (1983). *Interpreting children's drawings*. New York, NY: Brunner/Mazel.

Freud, A. (1967). *The ego and mechanisms of defense*. New York, NY: International Universities Press.

Freud, S. (1913). *The theory of interpretation of dreams*. New York, NY: Macmillan.

Freud, S. (1943). Remarks upon the theory and practice of dream-interpretation. *International Journal of Psychoanalysis, 24*(1–2), 66–71.

Grolnick, S. (1990). *The work and play of Winnicott*. Northvale, NJ: Jason Aronson.

Kohut, H., & Wolf, E. (1978). Disorders of the self and their treatment: An outline. *International Journal of Psychoanalysis, 59*, 413–425.

Kramer, E. (1971). *Art as therapy with children.* New York, NY: Schoken.

Luquet, G. H. (1913). *Les dessins d'un enfant: Etude psychologique.* Paris, France: Librairie Felix Alcan.

Maslow, A. (1967). *Toward a psychology of being.* Princeton, NJ: Van Nostrand.

Miller, A. (1981). *Prisoners of childhood.* New York, NY: Basic Books.

Piaget, J. (1954). *The construction of reality in the child.* New York, NY: Basic Books.

Rexford, E. (1978). *A developmental approach to problems of acting out.* New York, NY: International Universities Press.

Ullman, M., & Zimmerman, N. (1987). *Working with dreams.* London, England: Aquarian Press.

Weiser, J. (2010). Using photographs in art therapy practices around the world: Phototherapy, photo-art-therapy, and therapeutic photography. *Fusion* (a publication of Art Therapy Alliance, International Art Therapy Organization, and Art Therapy Without Borders), 2(3), 18–19.

Winnicott, D. W. (1960). Ego distortions in terms of true and false self. In D. W. Winnicott, *The maturational processes and the facilitating environment* (pp. 140–152). New York, NY: International Universities Press.

Winnicott, D. W. (1968). Playing: A theoretical statement. In D. W. Winnicott, *Playing and reality* (pp. 38–52). New York, NY: Tavistock.

Winnicott, D. W. (1971). *Playing and reality.* New York, NY: Tavistock.

Winnicott, D. W. (1975). Transitional objects and transitional phenomena. In D. W. Winnicott, *Through paediatrics to psychoanalysis* (pp. 229–242). New York, NY: Basic Books.

Wolf, R. (1976). The Polaroid technique: Spontaneous dialogues from the unconscious. *The International Journal of Art Psychotherapy, 3,* 197–214.

Wolf, R. (1978). Creative expressive therapy: An integrative case study. *The International Journal of Art Psychotherapy, 5,* 81–89.

Wolf, R. (1983). Instant phototherapy with children and adolescents. In D. Krauss & J. Fryrear (Eds.), *Phototherapy in mental health* (pp. 151–173). Springfield, IL: Charles C. Thomas.

Wolf, R. (1990). Visceral learning: The integration of aesthetic and creative process in education and psychotherapy. *Art Therapy: Journal of the American Art Therapy Association, 9,* 60–69.

Wolf, R. I. (2007). Advances in phototherapy training. *The Arts in Psychotherapy 34,* 124–133.

9

Poetry Therapy

Diane L. Kaufman, Rebecca C. Chalmers, and Wendy Rosenberg

INTRODUCTION

"The need to create is in every human being, and if that need is denied, life becomes distorted."

(Schneider, 1993, p. 43)

The healing power of poetic arts medicine is ancient in origin and encompasses body, mind, and spirit. According to poet Pat Schneider, MFA, founder and director emerita of Amherst Writers & Artists, so essential are poetic healing energies that our very life's unfolding may be damaged without creative self-expression. In Latin the word for poet is *vates* or "prophet." The Greek word, *poesis*, the origin of our word, poetry, literally means "to make or create." To the delight of countless children, the incantation "abracadabra" promises that upon utterance, amazing wonders will manifest. This magical word is of Aramaic origin and means, "I create as I speak." The National Association for Poetry Therapy states that in ancient Egyptian temples, the sick swallowed words written on papyrus prescribed as healing medicine (National Association for Poetry Therapy, History, n.d.). Spellbinding and enchanting, with an intensity of rhythm, image, sound, emotion, and meaning, poetic language becomes embodied and can serve as a metaphoric bridge to the divine, to within ourselves, and toward each other.

According to Greek mythology, Apollo was God of Medicine and Poetry. His son Ascepilus, born of a mortal woman, was the God of Healing (Hamilton, 1969). The Hippocratic Oath—the pledge of physicians to uphold the highest principles of their profession—opens with these words: "I swear by Apollo Physician and Asclepius and Hygieia and Panacea and all the gods and goddesses, making them my witnesses, that I will fulfill according to my ability and judgment this oath and this covenant." With lessons learned from antiquity, the Hippocratic Oath, which is still recited even today, serves as living witness and testimony to honor, uphold, and strengthen the triadic connection of poetry, medicine, and healing: the arts of medicine.

Pegasus, the flying horse, is the symbol of poetry in Greek mythology. Poseidon, the God of the Sea, and Medusa, the once-beautiful woman turned Gorgon by the Goddess Athena, conceived Pegasus. Because Medusa thought herself more beautiful than Goddess Athena, she was punished. She became so ugly that anyone who looked directly at her turned into stone. Athena ordered Perseus to kill Medusa. He was careful to look at Medusa only as a reflection in his shield. Out of Medusa's blood emerged Pegasus and his twin, the warrior Chrysaor, whose golden sword symbolized truth. It was said that whenever and wherever Pegasus struck his hoof, a wellspring of healing waters flowed. We still feel the presence of Pegasus when we look up at the constellation bearing his name (Hamilton, 1969; Mason, 1999).

A horse that flies? A golden sword? What does it all mean? And, if there is any meaning, a collective unconscious meaning, does it have anything to offer us here and now? Absolutely. According to Levine (1997), "the winged horse and the golden sword are auspicious symbols for the resources traumatized people discover in the process of vanquishing their own Medusas" (p. 66). Reclaiming the instinctual power of the body and the freedom of the creative mind, the trauma survivor can transform and heal. Engaging with poetry and the poetic in literature is like riding a horse bareback. Its spine supports you as you hug its ribs with your whole being.

How does poetry work its healing magic? To put it poetically:

Poetry rises to every occasion
Poetry honors all emotions and feelings
Poetry is a sacred place for words to gather
Poetry speaks out loud . . . or whispers in your ear
Poetry is a drawer you can pull open and unfold its contents
Poetry is a bicycle with handlebars you can grab onto and a
horn that beckons you to pay attention
Poetry is a way to communicate when talking doesn't suffice
Poetry reaches into places unreachable by other means
Poetry is words standing side by side holding hands
Poetry is words blowing in a field of tall grass
Poetry sits on the seat of your imagination
You can dig into your life with poetry

—Wendy Warren Rosenberg

POETRY THERAPY: PROCESS AND PROCEDURES

The process of making poems is a healing play: with words—
their sounds and shapes and associations; with time, as imagination breaks down barriers between past, present, and future;
and with emotional experience, the intuitive finding and communicating of things normally hidden. As children "play" this
game of poetry-making, they break through the limits of their
conscious, logical selves, and come to see self and world as freer,
more full of possibility, change, growth.
J.R. Michaels, PhD, Poet in the Schools for the
Geraldine R. Dodge Foundation and author
(personal communication, October 22, 2012)

Poetry therapy, sometimes referred to as bibliotherapy, creative writing therapy, or expressive writing therapy, is the purposeful use of literature to promote health and healing (Mazza, 2003). Poetry therapy is not
limited to poetry alone and can include many other modes of creative

verbal expression, such as stories, essays, journals, plays, songs, and movies. Poetry therapy can be used for nonclinical populations for personal growth and development and to ease symptoms and build skills for those receiving mental health services (Chavis & Weisberger, 2003). As a therapeutic intervention, poetry therapy draws out a child's creativity and imagination and can open up a recalcitrant teenager to share feelings. Poetry therapy can complement mental health treatment by enhancing insight (Reiter, 2009), encouraging behavioral change (Mazza, 2003), and increasing empathic connections (Fox, 1997). It may also benefit clinicians by supporting their own creativity and personal growth.

Poetry therapy includes a receptive component of reading and reflecting on writings and an expressive component of composing poems and other forms of creative verbal expression. Therapists can facilitate these poetic interventions with individuals, families, or groups. Poetry therapy can take place in the clinician's office, and the creative writing can continue in the child's home. What is written is not static or frozen in time, as there is always freedom to reflect anew and revise. In addition, and to great relief, this kind of expressive writing is not graded; there are no red marks here for errors in grammar or spelling. By bringing their truth into the world through the magic of word, image, rhythm, and sound, young authors become more self-aware, confident, and proud of themselves.

Poetry therapy is a dynamic process involving a triad of elements: the literature, the clinician, and the participant, in this case a child or adolescent (Hynes & Hynes-Berry, 2011). The creative verbal expression can serve as a catalyst for self-awareness, self-reflection, guided introspection, and deeper exploration through dialogue in therapy. According to Hynes and Hynes-Berry, the sensitive, skilled, and empathically attuned clinician introduces literature, not for academic but for therapeutic purposes. Poetry therapy is a means to encourage children's aliveness and responsiveness, promote better understanding of self and others, improve coping with reality, and ultimately foster children's overall emotional health and maturation.

History of Poetry Therapy as Therapy Modality

It was through the passionate efforts in the 1920s of Eli Griefer, a lawyer, pharmacist, and poet, and the psychiatrist Smiley Blanton that poetry began to emerge as a promising treatment modality in the United States (Hynes & Hynes-Berry, 2011). In the 1950s, Eli Griefer, in collaboration with psychiatrists Jack Leedy and Sam Spector, initiated the first poetry therapy group for psychiatric patients at Brooklyn's Cumberland Hospital (Leedy, 1969; Lerner, 1978). In 1969, Leedy founded the Association for Poetry Therapy (Leedy, 1985). In the 1970s, at Calabasas Neuropsychiatric Center, Arthur Lerner became Poet-in-Residence and Poetry Therapist and founded the Poetry Therapy Institute (National Association of Poetry Therapy, History, n.d.). Around the same time, librarian Arleen McCarty-Hynes partnered with psychiatrist Kenneth Gorelick to develop an in-depth poetry therapy training program at St. Elizabeth's Hospital in Washington, DC. The National Federation for Biblio/Poetry Therapy was incorporated in 1983 and serves as the training standards and credentialing agency (National Federation for Biblio/Poetry Therapy, n.d.). In 1981, the National Association for Poetry Therapy emerged from the Association for Poetry Therapy as a "community of healers" dedicated to promoting "growth and healing through language, symbol, and story" (National Association for Poetry Therapy, About, n.d.).

Theoretical Foundations of Poetry Therapy

In response to the question, "What makes a poem a poem?" Pat Schneider, MFA, replied: "It gives the reader a complete experience and it is language intensified" (1993, p. 107). Words are symbolic representations of the visible and invisible worlds we inhabit. Words are used to construct and explain the meaning of experiences and of our very existence. From infancy on, we are literally and figuratively spoon-fed and bathed in language, which can be viewed as a matrix through which we come to understand ourselves and our relationship with the world around us. From lullaby to nursery rhyme to fable and story, children are immersed in the power of poetic language, as it captures their attention through artful combination of playful sound, evocative imagery, and symbolic meaning. Poetry, when compared with all of the expressive arts, may be the most similar to the method of free association used in psychoanalysis. Both rely on the use of language, condensation, displacement, symbolization, and sublimation toward the aim of conflict resolution and problem solving (Robinson & Mowbray, 1985). This type of language deepens awareness. It enhances access to and expression of inner thoughts and feelings, and similar to psychotherapy, the process of poetry therapy can be an outlet, a catharsis for painful emotions. Through reading, writing, and discussing literature, new possibilities in thinking, feeling, and behaving can emerge.

Unlike traditional talk psychotherapy, therapeutic interventions in poetry therapy utilize reading and writing poems and stories to help create a safe distance and closeness from which children can explore thoughts and feelings that might otherwise be too dangerous or painful to express (Lengelle & Meijers, 2009). For example, children can express feelings of rage and despair through imagery and metaphor. Similarly, instead of engaging in maladaptive and acting-out behaviors, children can learn to communicate with their therapist through writing and meaningful conversation. As with psychotherapy, the writing and conversation is confidential and respectfully contained within the boundaries of the psychotherapy session. As Sherry Reiter, founder and director of The Creative "Righting" Center and author states:

> For children, metaphors in story and poetry bypass the natural resistance and provide safety from fear and other overwhelming emotions. We may create a story or poem to help a child with a particular conflict or challenge (prescriptive mode), or we may provide a child with support in co-creating a story or poem (expressive mode). By using animal characters, or sandtray figures, or personifying inanimate objects, a child's conflict can be replicated on a psychological level, and provide alternate solutions in a non-threatening way. The mind is naturally diverted and enchanted by metaphor, rhythm, rhyme and familiarity, so using these repetitiously informs the child in an entertaining way. (personal communication, November 25, 2012)

The facilitated dialogue about the poetic work includes spontaneous reflection on the poem's content and deeper meaning. Children may see familiar aspects of themselves in a poem and also what is unfamiliar, different, perhaps strange, and new. As a container for emotions that are common to humanity, reading and writing poetry in a therapeutic context reduces feelings of isolation and increases feelings of connection. Children are able to expand their view of the world while grasping the universal nature of many of their concerns. The positive outcome is enhanced empathy and emotional intelligence (Geraldine R. Dodge Poetry Festival, 2012).

"Writing poetry gives children permission to name the world as *they* see it without having to rename it for adults," says Tracy K. Smith, 2012 Pulitzer Prize Winner in Poetry (personal communication, October 17, 2012). Writing poetry validates and honors a child's inner world. Through listening to evocative language in poems and stories, reading to self or aloud to others, and writing imaginative stories and poems, children are helped to strengthen, express, and celebrate their own unique voices. Adolescents, in particular, struggle to consolidate their identity, which, according to Erikson, is the primary task of adolescent development (1968). Exploring new voices through the writing process can help adolescents develop a better understanding of themselves.

"Poetry is about wanting insight and believing you can find it" (Tracy K. Smith, personal communication, October 17, 2012). Belief, faith, and trust in the importance and inherent value of one's own being, of one's irreplaceable self and voice, and in the world being more safe and good than not, must be experienced and claimed by each child. As a foundation for self-esteem, this naming and renaming of one's self is vital. The practice of therapeutic writing affords the child unique opportunities to be known this way. Such focused writing also reinforces the conviction that life is worth examining and that we are able to learn from life's lessons. As Tracy K. Smith further explains, "A poem is a document of survival" (personal communication, October 17, 2012). The voice of the poet can testify to domination and cruelty on an individual and societal level. It can also testify to the truth that needs to be told. The poem's very creation testifies to the power of the human spirit and its determination to survive, thrive, and evolve.

Poetry Therapy, Mindfulness, and Other Therapy Approaches

Mindfulness-based techniques are used increasingly with children in the classroom, therapy offices, and other settings because they help children learn to regulate emotions, become curious about their minds, and improve attention and focus (Burke, 2010; Napoli, Krech, & Holley, 2004; Semple, Lee, & Miller, 2006). These techniques involve the conscious act of bringing one's attention to the present moment. Reading, reciting, and writing poetry are often incorporated into mindfulness-based practices; likewise, mindfulness-based techniques are often part of poetry therapy sessions.

The recitation of poems by children can mimic the mindfulness technique of deep breathing that leads to relaxation of body and mind. Children's verse and nursery rhymes are often highly rhythmic. Reading poems to children or asking them to read poetry aloud can be viewed as an artistic expression of the meditation facilitator's request to "follow your breath." The practice of writing is similar to meditation in that both promote relaxation, mindfulness, and focused attention. Because poetry is so rich in sensory imagery and metaphor, it naturally encourages children and adolescents to become more aware of their inner and outer worlds.

Writing about stressful or traumatic experiences and using poems to deepen awareness that allows for discussion of relevant concerns are examples of ways poetry therapy can be incorporated into other evidence-based therapies, such as cognitive processing therapy (CPT), cognitive therapy (Collins, Furman, & Langer, 2006), cognitive-behavioral therapy (CBT; Deblinger, Mannarino, Cohen, Runyon, & Steer, 2011), actualizing therapies, strength-based therapies (Furman, Pepi Downey, Jackson, & Bender, 2002), and narrative therapies (Smith, 1997). For example, CBT often uses expressive writing and poetry therapy techniques within and outside of therapy sessions toward restructuring maladaptive thoughts.

Research Support for Poetry Therapy

The impact of expressive writing on physical and mental health has attracted serious research. James W. Pennebaker and Sandra Beall (1986) found that among university students writing about stressful experiences, there was a long-term (six months) decrease in health problems. More than 20 years later in 2008, *The British Journal of Health Psychology* devoted an entire issue to research produced on the topic of expressive writing and health, citing that more than 200 studies on the topic had been published since the 1986 study (Smyth & Pennebaker, 2008). These studies cited benefits of expressive writing (particularly writing about stressful events) on health-related issues as varied as asthma, rheumatoid arthritis (Smyth, Stone, Hurewitz, & Kaell, 1999), immune system functioning (Pennebaker, Kiecolt-Glaser, & Glaser, 1988), and cancer (Low, Stanton, & Danoff-Burg, 2006). Similarly, expressive writing may improve mental health and behavioral disorders and related symptoms in conditions as diverse as sleep disorders and cognitive arousal leading to insomnia (Harvey & Farrell, 2003), mood disorders (Mooney, Espie, & Broomfield, 2009), and posttraumatic stress disorder (Smyth, Hockemeyer, & Tulloch, 2008). Despite the amount of research supporting the positive effects of expressive writing on health, Smyth and Pennebaker (2008) conclude that more research is indicated to help determine the specific writing-based interventions needed for a variety of populations and their particular health and mental conditions, as well as the mutative processes involved in expressive writing. This additional research could answer the question, *What exactly works for whom and why?*

Another body of research, qualitative and quantitative in nature, focuses on individual and group poetry therapy interventions among diverse populations including children and adolescents. In an article review on poetry therapy research conducted from 1969 to 2010, Heimes (2011) stated that "creative and therapeutic writing is increasingly used in the therapy, education, and advancement of children and young adults, in strengthening their feelings of self-esteem, in supporting their process of self-discovery, in facilitating communication and social integration, and in developing creative abilities as resources" (p. 2). Soliday, Garofalo, and Rogers (2004) found that an expressive writing intervention among adolescents generated increased optimism and decreased psychological distress. Another study found that adolescents who expressed emotions in writing about stressful events ("expressive writing") reported a greater decrease in anxiety compared to those who wrote about a neutral topic (Reynolds, Brewin, & Saxton, 2000). Poetry therapy has been shown to help adolescents and young adults grieve the death of a parent (Bowman, 1994), articulate conflicts, and manage aggression (Atlas, Smith, & Sessoms, 1992). It has also been shown to help special needs children improve their self-confidence and their sense of belonging (Olson-McBride & Page, 2006).

Limitations of Using Poetry Therapy

In utilizing poetry therapy to enhance therapeutic outcomes, certain guidelines are in order. Most importantly, the focus of treatment must always remain on the children. It must be remembered that the poem or other literature is a *therapeutic agent* in the skillful hands of the clinician. The poem is not an end in itself and is never a substitute for therapeutic acumen, skill, and training (Lerner, 1978). A poem can lead to intellectualization and withdrawal if the focus does not remain on the children's own responses and experiences. Another concern is when the clinician becomes overly invested in the literature itself, preferring the poem to the patient, and finds the relationship with the client has become secondary.

Poems must be chosen thoughtfully and for the therapeutic benefit of clients. Matching the emotional feel of poems to the moods of children, a term known as the *isoprinciple*, can help children recognize their emotions and normalize them (Leedy, 1985). However, the poems used in therapy must be chosen carefully, and the isoprinciple may not always be the best method of choice. For example, depressed young people's despair can be heightened with literature that matches their despondent mood, especially if it offers no positive solution. The clinician must also remain sensitive to the children's reading and writing level and choose appropriate literature and/or writing exercises. Poetry therapy is never a substitute for obtaining psychiatric evaluation, prescribing medication, or referring for hospitalization when necessary.

Children may on occasion bring in writing they claim as their own, when it was actually written by someone else. For example, an adolescent girl brought into a psychotherapy session "Phenomenal Woman" by Maya Angelou, with some discrete edits, saying she, herself, wrote the poem. Whereas in the school setting the emphasis would have focused on plagiarism, here the therapeutic approach was first to be sensitive to the teen's sense of self, to explore what had attracted her to the poem, to acknowledge that someone else had written the poem, and to encourage and empower her to honor and value her own creative voice.

The "borrowed" poem could then be used as a writing prompt or, alternatively, the teenager could write a letter to the published poet.

PRACTICAL TECHNIQUES AND CASE STUDIES

Integrating poetry therapy into clinical practice is facilitated by understanding a variety of poetry therapy techniques. In the following sections are examples of poetry therapy with individuals, families, and groups for children and adolescents.

Case Study 1

When I was preparing to lead one of my first poetry therapy groups, a 75-minute weekly group for adolescents at a drop-in homeless shelter in Washington, DC, I was concerned that poetry therapy would not connect with them. How would poetry and creative writing relate to teenagers? Would they be interested in such an academic word as *poetry* and even disdainful of expressing emotions in any situation that smacked of therapy? And how would this particular group of 14 teens—who were not only struggling with the typical storm and strife of the transition from childhood to adulthood but also with the instabilities of life's essentials such as shelter, money, food, and family—relate to a poem? Would they be able to see themselves in poetic language and be willing to write about and discuss their experiences?

I thought about this group that I had not yet met, these teens who had found themselves homeless by no choice of their own but by way of escape, rejection, and survival. What challenges might this group be facing as teens, and furthermore, as teens with few resources and often shattered families? The list of themes or schemas that might resonate with this group included:

- Having to survive on their own on the streets
- Having to separate from their families earlier than many teens
- Finding strength against difficult odds
- A desire and attempt to find a place to belong

I also made a list of developmental issues that teens in general might be grappling with, which included:

- Trying to formulate their identities, including what they value and what is important to them
- Yearning for independence
- Yearning for a sense of fitting in
- Experimentation and exploration
- Coping with intense emotions

Consider a poem that would speak to the issues that your group members may be facing. Some of the issues may be universal conflicts (e.g., struggling to overcome adversity) and some may be particular to a certain group (e.g., running away from an abusive home as a teen and adjusting to living in a homeless shelter). The poem "The Rose That Grew From Concrete," written by Tupac Shakur in his youth in the late 1980s before he became a famous rapper, seemed the perfect match with its accessible language and themes of hardships, abandonment, and resilience (Shakur, 1999).

Facilitate the Group

1. The Receptive Phase: Listening to the poem and discussion

The receptive/prescriptive component is the first part of the group that incorporates reading a poem to the group and inviting responses (Mazza, 1999). Typically, reading (or having individuals in the group read) a poem, short story, or excerpt from a memoir aloud and then silently is sufficient to elicit discussion. In this case, I found an audio recording of the poem that thoroughly engaged their attention.

"The Rose That Grew From Concrete" was released as a spoken-word track in 2000. In this recording, the poet Nikki Giovanni reads the poem in a strong and plain-spoken voice against a background of soulful instrumental music. I asked the group to take a deep breath and deeply listen to the song, letting the music and lyrics wash over them. We had a brief discussion about their visceral reactions to the piece: How does it make you feel? What is your experience as you listen to it?

I then passed out a copy of the poem, asked individuals to read it silently, and requested a volunteer to read it aloud. The young man who volunteered spoke in a booming and deep voice, which seemed surprising and out of sync for his slight stature. He appeared proud of his oration, and several members of the group noted how different his reading was from the recorded reading. The type of focused attention and observation elicited during this session is one example of how poems and the process of listening deeply to them can begin to encourage the practice of mindfulness.

After the group attended to the musicality of the poetic piece and how it affected them, I turned the discussion to the words and meaning of the work, starting with what might be literally happening in the poem, what it might metaphorically express, and then how it might relate to them personally. For this particular poem, which as the title suggests describes a rose remarkably surviving despite its hostile surroundings, I prepared the following discussion prompts (which could also be used for writing prompts):

- How are you like the rose?
- What are your dreams? How do you keep your dreams alive?
- Describe the concrete around you and how you grow in it.
- Have you ever felt like no one "even cared" as the last line of the poem suggests?

2. The Expressive Phase: Writing and Sharing

After individuals shared their ideas and feelings during the receptive/prescriptive part of the group, it was time for the expressive/creative component of the session (Mazza, 2003). Despite negative writing experiences they may have had in school, many of these adolescents were responsive to expressing themselves through writing. I encouraged group members to write whatever they pleased, reminding them that it did not have to rhyme or be in any specific form. I gave them the time frame (10 to 20 minutes) and asked group members who finished before the others to sit quietly and reflect. Some group members liked the free-writing format ("write whatever you're inspired to write"), whereas others preferred the structured prompt. I gave them the following writing prompts to choose from:

- Write your own poetic piece describing your life growing up in the city.
- Write about your dreams and how you plan to accomplish them.
- Write about when it felt like no one "even cared" and follow this with a time when someone did care and what this felt like.

After the writing time, I asked for volunteers to share their pieces. I modeled positive feedback, and then asked members to provide their own feedback. Peers often applauded and gave shouts of encouragement ("Yeah!") to group members who read their poems. Because teens yearn to be known for who they are and what they can do, the group's feedback had a beneficial effect on their self-worth. Sharing of writing was encouraged but not required. Listening carefully to other group members was a must.

3. Closure: Collaborative writing

To end this poetry therapy group session, I led a brief collaborative poem exercise. Collaborative, or group, poems have been shown to advance group cohesion and self-discovery more so than individual prescriptive poems (Golden, 2000). One approach to writing a collaborative poem is to ask group members to contribute individual responses to a common prompt.

For this particular group, I gave them a simple fill-in-the-blank prompt based on the original Shakur poem. The prompt was: "I am the rose that grows _____" and instructed each person to write down one to five words to finish the sentence. I acted as scribe, writing down each person's response, which culminated in a group poem. After reading their collaborative creation aloud, the group chose "Toward the Sun," one of the responses to the fill-in-the-blank exercise, as the poem's title. I typed the poem and distributed it to the group at the next session. The group members decided to display the collaborative poems from this session and future sessions on bulletin boards around the facility. The poetry therapy group helped these adolescents express their individual emotions and crystallize their identities while also helping them feel like they belonged to something bigger than themselves. They could pass by their group poems posted in the building and think, "I was a part of that."

Case Study 2

During a routine medication counseling session, I asked the twins, a girl and a boy who were both my patients, and their grandmother how they were doing, not just with their attention-deficit/hyperactivity disorder and symptom control, but how *they* were. The grandmother and children began to cry, and they expressed tremendous sadness over the death of their family pet. They were not only grieving the sudden loss of their cat, but they were also traumatized from witnessing their cat being killed by another animal.

I realized that the most important thing to do at that moment was to address on a deeper level the family's grief and loss, and knowing this, I put down my prescription pad. I asked the family to tell me stories about their cat. In hearing their heartfelt responses, I suggested to the family that their love for their cat and their cat's love for them could become a poem. The poem written in memory of Patches would be a testimony to love being more powerful than a brutal death. Their poem could replace the terrible images they had seen.

The acrostic poem, a simple poetry form, is created by starting each line with the first letters of a meaningful word or phrase. I wrote "PATCHES" down the left side of the paper and encouraged the family to share their feelings and memories about their pet. The first line began with a "P," the second, an "A," until the cat's full name was made into a poem. Afterward, the children and grandmother called their poem, "Patches We Love You." The children drew a picture and sang about their cat. The family took copies of the poem home with them.

Time passed and the family later agreed to be interviewed for an article about National Poetry Month and Poetry in Medicine Day at the University of Medicine and Dentistry of New Jersey. The grandmother shared with the reporter how poetry had helped her and the children. "I thought it was a good idea, because they could speak about how they felt about Patches. I framed it and put it in my house. Every now and then, we pick it up and read it. It helps to remember him" (Mascarenhas, 2010, p. 24). The most powerful and long-lasting medicine prescribed that day was poetry.

According to renowned storyteller Laura Simms, "Stories can render us interested in each other. When the story is a listening event between human beings, engaged and present, it accesses our inherent sources of healing and transformation" (personal communication, November 13, 2012). Another example of story and poetry therapy in my clinical practice took place during an initial assessment with a mother and daughter who had experienced the tragic loss of close family members in a fire. Although the traumatic event had happened years prior, it was immediately evident that the family was still grieving.

Continuing with the standard intake procedure seemed inappropriate. I would elicit this information, but the first priority was to focus on what was important. I needed to acknowledge the feelings in the room, respect the people who died, and acknowledge the survivors. I listened to mother and child recount the details of what happened. In listening to their lament, I recalled the myth of The Phoenix. I asked them if I could share with them this story and gave them the opportunity to say no. I explained that this was a made-up story and what had happened to them was real and terrible. As they were interested to know more, I printed out the myth, including images of the Phoenix. I shared with them that across all cultures were stories of this beautiful and magical bird. It lives for five hundred to a thousand years, and when it is time to die, it sets itself on fire. From its ashes arises the next Phoenix (New World Encyclopedia, n.d.). I reiterated that the fire in their lives was a tragic accident. I suggested that when horrific events happen, and there is destruction of meaning and making sense of the world, people have turned to the myth for comfort. I told them that children's author Hans Christian Andersen (1850), in his story about the Phoenix, suggested that the Phoenix was not a bird at all, but was really poetry. I asked them if they liked to write poetry, and the girl nodded. Soon her mother joined in. This is their poem:

The Phoenix

There is a phoenix in me
I will rise
Whenever I know
When the time is right

The sky will be bright
That way I will know
Everything will be all right
Because that's God in my sight

And He is letting you know
That with His Light
The time is right

Look at the light
Coming through the window
That way you will know
He is there for sure

While composing the poem, both mother and daughter exclaimed, "Look at the light coming through the window!" There were rays of sunlight suddenly shining on them. I suggested we add this to the poem. As the poem was written on Columbus Day, I shared with them, in the spirit of making meaning, that Christopher Columbus was searching for a new world. The mother replied, speaking of the poem-making experience, "The new world was always there, we only had to just find it." I suggested to the daughter that she could dedicate the poem if she liked, or not dedicate it, whatever seemed right for her. She decided to dedicate it to her loved ones who would "always be in our hearts." When the session ended, they asked for copies of their poem. We scheduled a follow-up session one week later to continue the intake. At that next session, they eagerly told me that they had shared with family members about the Phoenix myth and proudly showed them the poem they had written. They planned to ask family members to add more verses to the Phoenix poem. Myth was a powerful healing metaphor for this family, and their poem was a testimony to "rising from the ashes."

Case Study 3

Children may walk into the classroom carrying emotional baggage from home. Parents or siblings might have been arguing. Children may come to school without eating breakfast, having missed the bus, or be reacting to any number of other stressful circumstances that can impede learning. It may be easier to connect with these children through a creative approach. One technique I find useful is to have them read aloud and dramatize a poem such as Diane Stelling's "Sulking" (1997, p. 103):

Sulking

I'm so mad
I want to spit,
This is not
The end of it.
I was right,
And they were wrong,
I won't stay here
For very long.
No, I'll show them,
I'll make them cry,
I'll stay in here
Until I die.
They'll be sorry,
Wait and see,
They'll wish they hadn't
Punished me.
So even if
I'm here all night,
I'll prove my point –

I WAS RIGHT!

After children read aloud the poem one or more times, I follow up with questions such as: "How did that feel? Were there any lines you especially enjoyed saying? Were there any lines you didn't like hearing yourself say? Did the poem remind you of anything?" The responses can lead to further discussion. Suggesting that children use a word or phrase from "Sulking" to start their own poem can be a meaningful way for them to explore feelings.

CONCLUSION

Using poetry as a therapeutic intervention encourages a child to do more of and do better what a child does naturally: question, take risk, imagine and explore new possibilities, hug life and play! Adults often lose touch with poetry and become more "educated" which is to say more ensconced in mental frameworks that leave them barely capable of remembering that their imagination matters. Yet the healing poet within is natural and easier for a child to access—especially with the conscious support and appreciation of an adult who welcomes their creative expression. Poetic expression helps a child identify and find a place for feelings: loneliness, hurt, affection, wonder, the largeness of everything, fear of darkness, a longing to be seen and heard.

John Fox, CPT, founder and director of
The Institute for Poetic Medicine and author
(personal communication, November 21, 2012)

Even under the best of circumstances, growing up is not easy. This is even more likely when there are difficult family dynamics, traumatic experiences, or other stressful life events. Establishing and maintaining a therapeutic relationship between a troubled young person and a mental health practitioner can be challenging. Children or adolescents very often do not want to be in treatment, they minimize or deny having a problem, and they will assert their independence by not talking. Or, they may be limited in their skills to express and articulate, and be left feeling not understood, which in turn can leave the clinician feeling frustrated and ineffective. Creative approaches to therapy can be beneficial. Poetry therapy, with its emphasis on imagination, creativity, and verbal play taps into the natural abilities of children and can serve as a powerful healing intervention and resource.

Poetic arts medicine is alive and well, and Pegasus still flies!

SPECIALIZED TRAININGS AND RESOURCES

Major Organizations

The Geraldine R. Dodge Foundation
www.grdodge.org
Lapidus: Creative Words for Health and Well-Being
www.lapidus.org.uk

National Association for Poetry Therapy (NAPT)
www.poetrytherapy.org
National Federation for Biblio/Poetry Therapy
www.nfbpt.com

Relevant Websites

Amherst Writers and Artists
www.amherstwriters.com
Art Well
www.theartwell.org
The Center for Story and Symbol
www.folkstory.com
Favorite Poem Project
www.favoritepoem.org
Healing Story Alliance: Stories for Children in Crisis
www.healingstory.org/stories/crisis/index.html
Healing Words Productions
www.healingwordsproduction.com
International Academy for Poetry Therapy
www.iapoetry.org
Laura Simms: Storyteller, Writer, Humanitarian
www.laurasimms.com
Library of Congress Poetic Resources
www.loc.gov/rr/program/bib/1cpoetry
National Storytelling Network
www.storynet.org/index.html
Poetry Archive for Children
www.poetryarchive.org/childrensarchive/home.do
Poetry Foundation
www.poetryfoundation.org
Poetry 180: A Poem a Day for American High Schools
www.loc.gov/poetry/180
Poetry Out Loud
www.poetryoutloud.org
Poets House
www.poetshouse.org

Poets.org
    www.poets.org
Serious Play: Reading Poetry With Children
    www.poets.org/viewmedia.php/prmMID/17151
Teachers and Writers Collaborative
    www.twc.org
Transformative Language Arts Resource Center
    http://TLAresources.wordpress.com
Youth, Educators, and Storytellers Alliance
    www.yesalliance.org

Conferences

National Storytelling Network
    www.storynet.org/index.html
The Dodge Poetry Festival
    www.dodgepoetry.org
The National Association for Poetry Therapy
    www.napt.org

Trainings and Credentialing: Courses and Programs

The National Association for Poetry Therapy
    www.poetrytherapy.org/training.html
Center for Journal Therapy
    www.journaltherapy.com
International Academy for Poetry Therapy
    www.iapoetry.org
National Federation for Biblio/Poetry Therapy
    www.nfbpt.com
The Creative "Righting" Center
    http://users.erols.com/sreiter
The Institute of Poetic Medicine
    www.poeticmedicine.org

Audiovisual Resources

Children's Videos
    www.poetryfoundation.org/children/video

Geri Chavis
    www.jkp.com/blog/2011/07video-geri-chavis
John Fox on Open to Hope Radio
    www.youtube.com
Library of Congress Poetic Resources
    www.loc.gov/rr/program/bib/1cpoetry
Poetry Out Loud
    www.poetryoutloud.org/poems-and-performance/listen-to-poetry
Sherry Reiter Power of the Spoken Word
    www.youtube.com
Zur Institute: Cinema Therapy with Children and Adolescents
    www.zurinstitute.com/cinema_therapy_children_course.html

Books

Adams, K. (1990). *Journal to the self*. New York, NY: Warner Books.

Boulton, G., Field, V., & Thompson, K. (Eds.). (2006). *Writing works: A resource handbook for therapeutic writing workshops and activities*. London, England: Jessica Kingsley.

Brooke, S. L (Ed.). (2006). *Creative arts therapies manual: A guide to the history, theoretical approaches, assessment, and work with special populations of art, play, dance, music, drama, and poetry therapies*. Springfield, IL: Charles C. Thomas.

Chavis, G. G. (2011). *Poetry and story therapy: The healing power of creative expression*. Philadelphia, PA: Jessica Kingsley.

Fletcher, R. (2002). *Poetry matters: Writing a poem from the inside out*. New York, NY: Harper Trophy.

Fox, J. (1995). *Finding what you didn't lose: Expressing your truth and creativity through poem-making*. New York, NY: Jeremy P. Tarcher/Putnam.

Ganim, B. (1999). *Art and healing: Using expressive art to heal your body, mind, and spirit*. New York, NY: Three Rivers Press.

Heard, G. (1999). *Awakening the heart: Exploring poetry in elementary and middle school*. Portsmouth, NH: Heinemann.

Janeczko, P. B. (Ed.). (2002). *Seeing the blue between: Advice and inspiration for young poets*. Somerville, MA: Candlewick Press.

Koch, K., & Padgett, R. (1999). *Wishes, lies, and dreams*. New York, NY: HarperCollins.

Manjusvara. (2010). *The poet's way*. Cambridge, UK: Windhorse Publications.

Michaels, J. R. (1999). *Risking intensity: Reading and writing poetry with high school students*. Urbana, IL: National Council of Teachers of English.

Miller, R. (2008). *Dance with the elephants: Free your creativity and write.* Sarasota, FL: Robi Jode Press.

Morice, D. (1995). *The adventures of Dr. Alphabet: 104 unusual ways to write poetry in the classroom and the community.* New York, NY: Teachers and Writers Collaborative.

Morrison, M. (Ed.). (1987). *Poetry as therapy.* New York, NY: Human Science Press.

Padgett, R. (Ed.). (2000). *The teachers and writers handbook of poetic forms.* New York, NY: T&W Books.

Pennebaker, J. W. (1997). *Opening up: The healing power of expressing emotions.* New York, NY: Guilford Press.

Simms, L. (2011). *Our secret territory: The essence of story-telling.* Boulder, CO: Sentient Publications.

Stelling, D. (1999). *The giant and the mouse.* Butler, NJ: Hereami Publishing.

Therrien, R. (1999). *Voices from the 'hood: How to start and sustain a writing workshop for youth at risk.* Amherst, MA: Amherst Writers & Artists Press.

Woodward, P. (1996). *Journal jumpstarts: Quick topics and tips for journal writing.* Fort Collins, CO: Cottonwood Press.

Woolridge, S. G. (1996). *Poemcrazy: Freeing your life with words.* New York, NY: Clarkson Potter.

The Journal of Poetry Therapy (Fall 1987 to present) is the primary source of current articles, resources, news, abstracts of articles from other journals, dissertation abstracts, and original poetry.

The Museletter, published three times per year, is the official newsletter of the National Association for Poetry Therapy.

REFERENCES

Andersen, H. C. (1850). The phoenix bird. Retrieved from http://www.hca.gilead.org.il/phoenix.html

Atlas, J. A., Smith, P., & Sessoms, L. (1992). Art and poetry in brief therapy of hospitalized adolescents. *The Arts in Psychotherapy, 19*(4), 279–283.

Bowman, D. O. (1994). The application of poetry therapy in grief counseling with adolescents and young adults. *Journal of Poetry Therapy, 8*(2), 63–73.

Burke, C. A. (2010). Mindfulness-based approaches with children and adolescents: A preliminary review of current research in an emergent field. *Journal of Child and Family Studies, 19*(2), 133–144.

Chavis, G. G., & Weisberger, L. L. (Eds.). (2003). *The healing fountain: Poetry therapy for life's journey.* St. Cloud, MN: North Star Press.

Collins, K. S., Furman, R., & Langer, C. L. (2006). Poetry therapy as a tool of cognitively based practice. *The Arts in Psychotherapy, 33*, 180–187.

Deblinger, E., Mannarino, A. P., Cohen, J. A., Runyon, M. K., & Steer, R. A. (2011). Trauma-focused cognitive behavioral therapy for children: The impact of the trauma narrative and treatment length. *Depression and Anxiety, 28*, 67–75.

Erikson, E. H. (1968). *Identity: Youth and crisis.* New York, NY: W. W. Norton.

Fox, J. (1997). *Poetic medicine: The healing art of poem-making.* New York, NY: Jeremy P. Tarcher/Putnam.

Furman, R., Pepi Downey, E., Jackson, R. L., & Bender, K. (2002). Poetry therapy as a tool for strengths-based practice. *Advances in Social Work, 3*(2), 146–157.

Geraldine R. Dodge Poetry Festival. (2012). Festival kit for teachers. Butler, NJ: The Geraldine R. Dodge Foundation.

Golden, K. M. (2000). The use of collaborative writing to enhance cohesion in poetry therapy groups. *Journal of Poetry Therapy, 13*(3), 125–136.

Hamilton, E. (1969). *Mythology.* New York, NY: New American Library.

Harvey, A. G., & Farrell, C. (2003). The efficacy of a Pennebaker-like writing intervention for poor sleepers. *Behavioral Sleep Medicine, 1*(2), 115–124.

Heimes, S. (2011). State of poetry therapy research (review). *The Arts in Psychotherapy, 38*, 1–8.

Hynes, A., & Hynes-Berry, M. (2011). *Biblio/poetry therapy: The interactive process: A handbook* (3rd ed.). St. Cloud, MN: North Star Press.

Leedy, J. J. (Ed.). (1969). *Poetry therapy: The use of poetry in the treatment of emotional disorders.* Philadelphia, PA: J. B. Lippincott.

Leedy, J. J. (Ed.). (1985). *Poetry as healer: Mending the troubled mind.* New York, NY: Vanguard Press.

Lengelle, R., & Meijers, F. (2009). Mystery to mastery: An exploration of what happens in the black box of writing and healing. *Journal of Poetry Therapy, 22*(2), 57–75.

Lerner, A. (Ed.). (1978). *Poetry in the therapeutic experience.* New York, NY: Pergamon Press.

Levine, P. (1997). *Waking the tiger: Healing trauma.* Berkeley, CA: North Atlantic Books.

Low, C. A., Stanton, A. L., & Danoff-Burg, S. (2006). Expressive disclosure and benefit finding among breast cancer patients: Mechanisms for positive health effects. *Health Psychology, 25*(2), 181–189.

Mascarenhas, R. (2010, April 29). NJ scholars say poetry therapy can improve patients' emotional health. *Star Ledger,* 24.

Mason, J. (1999). *The flying horse: The story of pegasus.* New York, NY: Grosset & Dunlap.

Mazza, N. (1999). *Poetry therapy: Interface of the arts and psychology.* Boca Raton/London: CRC Press.

Mazza, N. (2003). *Poetry therapy: Theory and practice.* New York, NY: Brunner-Routledge.

Mooney, P., Espie, C. A., & Broomfield, N. M. (2009). An experimental assessment of a Pennebaker writing intervention in primary insomnia. *Behavioral Sleep Medicine, 7,* 99–105.

Napoli, M., Krech, P. R., & Holley, L. C. (2004). Mindfulness training for elementary school students: The attention academy. *Journal of Applied School of Psychology, 21*(1), 99–125.

National Association for Poetry Therapy. (n.d.). About the National Association for Poetry Therapy. Retrieved from www.poetrytherapy.org/index.html

National Association for Poetry Therapy. (n.d). History. Retrieved from www.poetrytherapy.org/history.html

National Federation for Biblio/Poetry Therapy. (n.d.). History of the Federation. Retrieved from www.nfbpt.com/history.html

New World Encyclopedia. (n.d.). Phoenix (mythology). Retrieved from http://newworldencyclopedia.org/entry/Phoenix

Olson-McBride, L., & Page, T. (2006). Poetry therapy with special needs children: A pilot project. *Journal of Poetry Therapy, 19,* 167–183.

Pennebaker, J. W., & Beall, S. K. (1986). Confronting a traumatic event: Toward an understanding of inhibition and disease. *Journal of Abnormal Psychology, 95*(3), 274–281.

Pennebaker, J. W., Kiecolt-Glaser, J., & Glaser, R. (1988). Disclosure of traumas and immune function: Health implications for psychotherapy. *Journal of Consulting and Clinical Psychology, 56,* 239–245.

Reiter, S. (Ed.). (2009). *Writing away the demons: Stories of creative coping through transformational writing.* St. Cloud, MN: North Star Press.

Reynolds, M., Brewin, C. R., & Saxton, M. (2000). Emotional disclosure in school children. *Journal of Child Psychology and Psychiatry, 41,* 151–159.

Robinson, S. S., & Mowbray, J. K. (1985). Why poetry? In J. J. Leedy (Ed.), *Poetry as healer: Mending the troubled mind* (pp. 17–27). New York, NY: Vanguard Press.

Schneider, P. (1993). *The writer as an artist: A new approach to writing alone and with others.* Los Angeles, CA: Lowell House.

Semple, R. J., Lee, J., & Miller, L. F. (2006). Mindfulness-based cognitive therapy for children. In R. A. Baer (Ed.), *Mindfulness-based treatment approaches:*

Clinician's guide to evidence base and applications (pp. 143–165). Oxford, UK: Academic Press/Elsevier.

Shakur, T. (1999). *The rose that grew from concrete: Poems.* New York, NY: Pocketbooks/Simon & Schuster.

Smith, C. (1997). Introduction: Comparing traditional therapies with narrative approaches. In C. Smith & D. Nylund (Eds.), *Narrative therapies with children and adolescents* (pp. 1–47). New York, NY: Guilford Press.

Smyth, J. M., Hockemeyer, J. R., & Tulloch, H. (2008). Expressive writing and post-traumatic stress disorder: Effects on trauma symptoms, mood states, and cortisol reactivity. *British Journal of Health Psychology, 13,* 85–93.

Smyth, J. M., & Pennebaker, J. W. (2008). Exploring the boundary conditions of expressive writing: In search of the right recipe. *British Journal of Health Psychology, 13*(1), 1–7.

Smyth J. M., Stone, A. A., Hurewitz, A., & Kaell, A. (1999). Effects of writing about stressful experiences on symptom reduction in patients with asthma or rheumatoid arthritis: A randomized trial. *Journal of the American Medical Association, 281*(14), 1304–1309.

Soliday, E., Garofalo, J. P., & Rogers, D. (2004). Expressive writing intervention for adolescents' somatic symptoms and mood. *Journal of Clinical Child and Adolescent Psychology, 3*(4), 792–801.

Stelling, D. (1997). *One little voice.* Butler, NJ: Hereami Publishing.

10

Integrating Play and Expressive Art Therapy Into Educational Settings: A Pedagogy for Optimistic Therapists

Jodi M. Crane and Jennifer N. Baggerly

INTRODUCTION TO CREATIVE EXPERIENTIAL LEARNING

Creative Experiential Learning (CEL) is an educational method that involves interactive, collaborative, multimodal learning through seeing, hearing, talking, and doing, which leads to a better retention and understanding of information (Gibson, 2010; Guevara, 2002; Vernon & Tollerud, 2001). CEL is a type of active learning that involves students in *doing* things and *thinking about* the things they are doing (Bonwell & Eison, 1991). The rationale is based on Dale's (1969) seminal research, which indicates that after two weeks, people remember 10% of what they read, 20% of what they hear, 30% of what they see, 50% of what they see and hear, 70% of what they say, and 90% of what they say and do.

During the CEL process, students engage in an activity or manipulate materials; explore, reflect, and discover connections; make meaning from the activity; and then apply what was learned (Deaver & Shiflett, 2011; Ogunleye, 2002; Warren, Zavaschi, Covello, Zakaria, 2012). Rather than encouraging passive learning, CEL is a social constructivist approach in which students create their own knowledge and meaning through interaction with each other (McAuliffe & Eriksen, 2011). CEL involves "repeated opportunities to observe, debate, reflect and practice" (Larson, 2004, p. 19). Hence, students are more likely to achieve higher orders of learning, such as application, evaluation, and synthesis of concepts (Baggerly, 2002).

CEL assumes that everyone has the inherent capacity or seeds to be creative (i.e., to create something meaningful and useful). It is a myth that one either is creative or is not (Edelson, 1999; Henshon, 2009). Creativity includes the person, process, and product of the creative endeavor and can comprise novelty, play, spontaneity, and innovation (Bleakley, 2004; Kleiman, 2008). Therefore, "the ultimate question, then, is not how to teach creativity, but rather how to understand, harvest, and build up the very creativity that every student already possesses and uses" (Livingston, 2010, p. 61). This optimistic view of students motivates the teacher to value contributions from all.

CEL requires instructors to forego the traditional educational process of lecturing during most of the class time. Lecturing may seem easier for some instructors because it is familiar to them. Yet, research in higher education settings shows that students only pay attention to a lecture an average of 15 minutes (Bonwell & Eison, 1991). CEL instructors must value the students more than the curriculum (Ballon, Silver, & Fidler, 2007). Instructors must give up the tyranny of the content for the value of integrated learning. This requires instructors to embrace a paradigm shift from being the "sage on the stage" to being the "guide on the side" (Bonwell & Eison, 1991). Because designing CEL activities can be time consuming (Vernon & Tollerud, 2001), instructors can remind themselves of the words of child-centered play therapy expert Garry Landreth, "Folks, if it's important we should take time for it" (Center for Play Therapy, 1994).

Benefits of CEL

CEL has both personal and professional benefits for students in training programs related to the expressive art therapies. First, creative activities facilitate self-expression and openness, because intellectual ego defenses are bypassed and powerful images are accessed. For example, asking students to select a miniature animal (toy or picture) that reflects their self-image yields a deeper self-expression and openness than verbally stating their self-image.

Second, reflection of the creative process can lead to self-awareness and self-acceptance. A product made or selected during an activity can become a visual reminder of what was learned (Guevara, 2002). If a student selects a toy elephant to represent herself, she may become aware that she feels conspicuous about her weight but come to a newfound appreciation of her strength.

Third, CEL group discussions can result in empathy and problem solving. Seeing and hearing that a student selected an elephant because of insecurities about weight may help students empathize with others who feel conspicuous. Problem solving is enhanced by using the creative right side of the brain. For example, the group could generate problem-solving ideas by discussing how the other animals could help the elephant feel more comfortable.

Fourth, because CEL activities are often fun and relaxing, they support self-care and wellness (Deaver & Shiflett, 2011; Warren et al., 2012; Ziff & Beamish, 2004). Finally, CEL gives students direct experiential knowledge about the advantages and limits of the expressive arts and play therapy (Deaver & Shiflett, 2011; Dunn-Snow & Joy-Smellie, 2000; Ziff & Beamish, 2004). This direct knowledge provides students with needed confidence to lead their own clients through the expressive art and play activities.

PREPARATION

Instructor Preparation

Instructor preparation for CEL entails developing several general pedagogical skills. General pedagogical skills begin with the ability to create a positive and trusting environment. Instructors can set a positive tone by sharing their passion for expressive arts and play therapy. Creating a trusting environment where students do not feel manipulated or tricked is also important (Ballon et al., 2007). This is accomplished by explicitly stating activity objectives, such as increasing self-awareness to mitigate counter-transference. Explaining the rationale for the social constructionist CEL approach, as described previously, will facilitate students' commitment to the method.

Engaging students is another general pedagogical skill. To engage students, instructors must model the very things they are requesting of their students, specifically risk taking, open-mindedness, imagination, and comfort with self-expression. For example, they can share their own initial hesitation with an activity and how their persistence resulted in self-awareness of a personal barrier. Instructors can also engage students by inviting them to examine assumptions and investigate issues from a variety of perspectives (Boldt & Paul, 2011; Gibson, 2010). Another method of engaging students is by varying voice, rhythm, pace, activities, and class structure and assignments (Grainer, Barnes, & Scoffham, 2004). Instructors can support student attention by moving about the room, in and among the students at different times throughout the class. However, too much change can leave students feeling anxious and insecure.

Facilitating discussions is another core pedagogical skill. Instructors need to pose specific, open-ended questions rather than general questions. For example, rather than asking, "Did this activity make sense to you?" instructors can present several different case scenarios and ask students to form small groups to discuss how they would explain the rationale for an activity to each client.

In addition to specific questions, discussion starters include elaborating on a specific quotation from the reading, contrasting differing perspectives, considering societal impact, and debating ethical dilemmas. In order to engage all students in the discussion, instructors can use the strategy of "think, pair, share," in which students first write their response and then share their writing with a fellow student (Baggerly, 2002). To prevent dominance by one student, instructors can ask students from the opposite side of the classroom to respond first. If needed, instructors can privately suggest to overly dominant students that they try a new skill of first listening to other students' contributions before sharing their view.

Pacing is a needed general pedagogical skill. CEL instructors must balance structure with flexibility while paying attention to the timing and pacing of delivery. It is important to discern when to sensitively approach opportunities for personal application and when to withdraw or create distance (Bleakley, 2004; Gibson, 2010). For example, if class time is ending in 10 minutes, then instructors need to encourage students to journal about their personal insights rather than probing deeper into the issue at the end of class. Instructors also need to be aware that too much evaluation, competition, pressure, and limited choices can stifle creativity (Gibson, 2010; Hargreaves, 2008).

Conflict management is another key pedagogical skill (Grainer et al., 2004; Larson, 2004). Instructors should exhibit that they are comfortable with ambiguity and tolerant of differing views. When conflicts arise, they convey confidence that students have something valuable to offer each other and encourage students to expand their thinking and sensing so learning can occur (Clegg, 2008; Hargreaves, 2008; Vernon & Tollerud, 2001). By doing so, instructors will role model that they are self-assured and lifelong learners who glean knowledge even during conflicts (Grainer et al., 2004). When a controversial view or action arises, instructors ask students to pause and think of a constructive way to share their view or research-based information.

The final pedagogical skill is to maintain ethical principles and boundaries. CEL instructors respect students' autonomy, avoid harm (nonmaleficence), and ensure student well-being (Hargreaves, 2008). They must provide boundaries so relationships with students do not become that of therapists and clients (Ziff & Beamish, 2004). Instructors should know ahead of time how to support those who become emotional during an activity, uncover buried trauma, or reveal more than they intended (Deaver & Shiflett, 2011; Jones, 1992). Instructors can process with students individually after class time or make a referral for counseling if necessary.

In addition to these general pedagogical skills, play and expressive art therapy instructors need ongoing continuing education in the arts and play therapy. This preparation can be accomplished by attending conferences or workshop trainings and viewing training videos. Training conferences and materials are available from the Association for Play Therapy at http://www.a4pt.org and the American Art Therapy Association at http://arttherapy.org to name a couple of websites. Instructors should experience each expressive art and play therapy activity themselves before engaging students in the activity (Hargreaves, 2008). Doing so allows instructors time to identify positive outcomes, such as appreciation of differing perspectives (e.g., a family art therapy activity), and to prepare for possible negative outcomes, such as paint splattered on clothing or anger splashed on a previously held perfect perception of family.

Physical Preparation

The physical learning environment should include enough space so students can comfortably move around and interact with one another. It is helpful for the classroom to have tables for group work; open space for drama, movement, and role play; a sink nearby for cleanup of art materials; and electronic equipment for audiovisual materials (Edelson, 1999; Ziff & Beamish, 2004). In addition, expressive arts and play activities may be more easily performed when there is soft lighting; blankets, pillows, and carpet squares for the floor; and nonlyrical music (Jones, 1992). Instructors can set the mood for various activities by lowering lights and playing meditative music (Deaver & Shiflett, 2011; Guevara, 2002).

Student Preparation

CEL may be a new approach for students who are used to the traditional model of lecture and note-taking. Instructors need to encourage students to take ownership of their learning by being active learners rather than passive recipients. Instructors can ask students how they learn best and invite feedback on how they envision the structure of the class and their contribution to it (Gibson, 2010; Vernon & Tollerud, 2001). Doing so will help students be invested in their learning and embrace the social constructionist approach. Informing students that they will be challenged to engage, reflect, and explore answers for themselves will prevent them from being overly dependent on the instructor (Grainer et al., 2004; Ogunleye, 2002).

Instructors can also prepare students by anticipating and addressing their initial resistance. Some students may seem shy or resistant, voice a dislike for the activity, or say things like, "I can't draw." They may appear self-conscious, judgmental of the quality of their work, or edit themselves (Guevara, 2002; Warren et al., 2012; Ziff & Beamish, 2004). Sometimes this difficulty suggests issues they are dealing with personally (Boldt & Paul, 2011). These reactions are also more likely to be seen in students with previous art-related learning experiences for which they were judged harshly. For some, their experiences are like a wound that has not healed. Instructors can verbalize this possibility and ask students to compartmentalize previous judgments by writing them down and sealing them in an envelope.

CEL activities often involve risk, which leads to fear of the unknown, failure, or ridicule (Hargreaves, 2008). Students may feel intimidated if they are not used to expressing themselves in artistic ways (Ziff & Beamish, 2004), and they may feel that what they made is too personal to share (Deaver & Shiflett, 2011). Instructors can remind students that much of human experience involves some level of vulnerability. As vulnerability researcher Brené Brown (2010) stated, "staying vulnerable is a risk we have to take if we want to experience connection" (p. 53).

The antidote to fear is encouragement and trust. Wise CEL instructors take the necessary time to build good relationships with their students and the students with one another via simple, nonthreatening activities, such as making spontaneous images from a scribble, magazine clippings, or paint (Malchiodi, 2007). Students might also be given a straightforward prompt, such as to paint their feelings. One student who was instructed to paint her feelings stuck her brush into the tempera paint and quickly jabbed the paper, resulting in brown blobs all over the page. The student verbally shared with her small group that she was experiencing morning sickness. Group members then empathized with her, and she seemed more relaxed as a consequence. Malchiodi's (2007) *The Art Therapy Sourcebook* is an excellent resource for introducing students to the therapeutic use of art materials.

Instructors can also prepare students for activities by varying the size of groups depending on the activity. For activities that require art or personal sharing, small groups can help students work through inhibition and lack of confidence. For activities that require performance, large groups help students feel more secure. For example, most students feel more comfortable when singing all together in a large group.

PROCESS

Throughout the process, CEL instructors engage in informed consent, formative assessment, variation in methods and media, continual encouragement, and processing and debriefing. The following sections describe these components.

Informed Consent

Before beginning an activity in class, instructors need to provide informed consent about the activity's purpose, time commitment, process, intended outcomes, and possible risks (Dunn-Snow & Joy-Smellie, 2000; Jones, 1992). This information helps students know what to expect so they can make an informed decision about their level of participation. For example, if an activity's purpose is to explore students' view of loss, students who have had a recent significant loss may feel too vulnerable to participate. Instructors need to respect students' right to autonomy by not pressuring them to participate in an activity. Instructors can invite students to participate in something out of their comfort zones as long as they also communicate they will maintain respect for students who decline (Boldt & Paul, 2011; Deaver & Shiflett, 2011).

Instructors should reassure students that the goal is to maintain a safe, nonjudgmental environment. To prevent ridicule, instructors can remind students to be respectful and not to make fun of one another (Dunn-Snow & Joy-Smellie, 2000; Guevara, 2002). It is also important to reassure students that it is okay to fail, because expertise is not the goal (Grainer et al., 2004; Larson, 2004; Ziff & Beamish, 2004).

Assessment

In line with the philosophy of CEL, instructors use formative, authentic, ongoing assessment to continually evaluate and improve their instruction (Gibson, 2010). This type of assessment can involve students and be integrated into the learning process. For example, students could devise a rubric to be used to assess basic play therapy skills. Personal portfolios also allow students to demonstrate their learning in a creative way that provides a permanent product for future reflection.

Variation in Methods and Media

Instructors can use a variety of methods and media to stimulate students' interest. Virtual or real-life field trips to play therapy rooms, theatres, and art, photography, or music studios can inspire students. Guest speakers can be particularly useful to help students learn material with which the instructor does not have expertise (Boldt & Paul, 2011). Furthermore, instructors can incorporate a range of media that engage students visually, cognitively, and emotionally. Video clips from popular films, Internet videos, props, diagrams, photos, artwork, metaphors, stories and anecdotes, lyrical music, and items from nature can be used to illustrate important concepts as well as personalize the instructor's teaching (Grainer et al., 2004; Guevara, 2002; Vernon & Tollerud, 2001).

Manipulatives can also stimulate students' interest. A small container of Play-Doh, for example, can help students retrieve childhood memories when instructors ask students to close their eyes, open the container, and smell its contents. A baby mobile can be used to demonstrate the family system's concept of mutual, reciprocal influence, that what happens to one family member affects the rest of the family. A pair of rose-colored glasses and a pair of grey-colored glasses can be used to demonstrate the concept of family members having multiple perspectives on an issue (Vernon & Tollerud, 2001).

In order to alleviate students' insecurities about their limited artistic or creative abilities, instructors can read children's books to the class. The books *The Dot* and *Ish* by Peter Reynolds, *Not a Box* and *Not a Stick* by Antoinette Portis, *Beautiful Oops!* by Barney Saltzberg, and *Harold and the Purple Crayon* by Crockett Johnson serve these purposes.

Sharing excerpts from novels can also exemplify important concepts. For instance, in helping students understand Virginia Axline's (1947) play therapy principle of accepting the child completely, the first author (Crane) reads a portion from Martha Beck's (1999) memoir *Expecting Adam*. In this section, Beck describes going for a run as an undergraduate student and spotting a beautiful piece of rose quartz on the ground. When she picks it up, she sees that it is actually a piece of Styrofoam and drops it, disgusted. She realizes that her two labels for the object influenced her reaction to it. Later that evening, she attempts an experiment of trying not to ascribe any labels to her fellow students as they file through the dining hall line. However, she stopped the experiment. Beck wrote, "I was so overcome by the beauty of every person in that dining hall that my eyes kept filling with tears. I think that's why we screen out so much loveliness. If we saw people as they really are, the beauty would overwhelm us" (p. 322).

Continual Encouragement

CEL instructors consistently give students descriptive praise, encouragement, and constructive feedback throughout the entire class. Doing so motivates and engages students in their learning, whereas not doing so can lead to apathy and lack of participation (Grainer et al., 2004). For instance, if instructors respond to student comments and questions by acknowledging their desire to learn and affirming at least one aspect of their comment, then other students are motivated to contribute. For example: "Your question shows you are learning to distinguish between praise and encouragement. I like your description of praise. Let's add . . ." In contrast, if instructors respond with criticism, then students are less likely to contribute to class discussion.

Another way to encourage students in learning is by seeing their instructors demonstrate expressive arts and play therapy with an actual client (Larson, 2004). This method can easily be accomplished by showing a video of a client session (if consent is obtained).

Processing and Debriefing

Instructors must ensure there is enough time to reflect, debrief, and process after an activity (Ballon et al., 2007; Boldt & Paul, 2011).

The goal of processing is for students to apply what they have learned. Processing can be facilitated by using open-ended questions such as, "How has today's activity impacted you?" or "What would happen if . . . ?" or "One thing I learned about myself, others, and the world is . . ." (Grainer et al., 2004; Ogunleye, 2002). During the processing period, instructors need to keep students on track instead of straying off topic. At the end of the class, instructors can ask students to synthesize what was shared (Guevara, 2002). Students can continue processing by sharing their reactions through electronic means (e.g., e-mail, online discussion boards; Vernon & Tollerud, 2001). Journaling can also facilitate deeper processing. Instructors can encourage students to journal their self-reflection and self-observation as well as thoughts and feelings before, during, and after an activity (Larson, 2004). Expressive arts may also be incorporated into the journal through drawings, collages, poems, and photographs. Journaling can even be done through verbalizing into a voice recorder such as a smartphone (Vernon & Tollerud, 2001).

ACTIVITIES

Warm-Up Activities

The beginning activity in a class sets the tone and prepares students for deeper activities. Quotes, poems, and comic strips can be used to introduce a theme or to illustrate important points. *Calvin and Hobbes* by Bill Watterson, *For Better or For Worse* by Lynn Johnson, *One Big Happy* by Rick Detorie, *The Family Circus* by Bil and Jeff Keane, and, of course, *Peanuts* by Charles Schulz all contain delightful child characters. Books by Fred Rogers (2003, 2006) contain many quotations that fit with the philosophy of humanistic play therapy. After sharing the opening quote, poem, or comic strip, the instructor asks students to elaborate on how the message informs students' view of self, children, or the therapy process.

Another warm-up activity for the beginning of class is to have students take five minutes to answer a question about their childhood with a classmate (Vernon & Tollerud, 2001). For example, "What was a childhood experience that shaped your view of people from other

Figure 10.1   The Play Assessement

By Dr. Jodi Crane

To work successfully with children, you must first be comfortable with the world of childhood. To facilitate this, it is important to assess your own attitude about play and playfulness. Reflect on your childhood as best as you remember as you answer these questions:

1. FAMILY'S ATTITUDE

   Describe your family's attitude about play when you were a child.
   - What were your parents' reactions to your play? Include any restrictions on play (e.g., location, amount of noise, messiness, etc.).
   - Did your parents play with you? If so, what, and how often?
   - What types of fun or playful activities did your family enjoy together?

2. YOUR TYPICAL PLAY

   Describe in detail your typical play as a child. Include:
   - Where you played
   - Who you played with (e.g., Did you prefer to play alone or with siblings, friends, or relatives and did you have an imaginary playmate?)
   - What you did (your favorite play activities) including games (e.g., physically active, board, card, or solitary), make-believe/pretend play and role you tended to play, use of imaginary heroes (e.g., Superman, Indiana Jones, Han Solo)
   - Your favorite toy(s) and why it was your favorite

3. BOOKS

   Describe your family's attitude toward reading.
   - Were you read to as a child? If so, by whom? What was this experience like?
   - What was (were) your favorite book(s) as a child? Why?

4. PETS

   Describe your favorite childhood pet.
   - What did this pet mean to you?

5. CURRENT ATTITUDE

   Describe your current attitude toward play.
   - How do you play now as an adult?
   - Who or what has most influenced your current attitudes about play? How?

6. THIS EXPERIENCE

   Describe what this experience has been like for you.
   - What memories or feelings were evoked as you completed this exercise?
   - What did you learn from this experience?
   - What can you tap into from your own childhood experiences to carry with you into your adult world as you work with children?

Adapted from C. F. Sori (2003).

countries?" or "My parents' style of discipline communicated that I was (fill in the blank)." To increase a sense of class community, students share with a new classmate each time. Crane expanded on Vernon and Tollerud's activity by developing *The Play Assessment* (see Figure 10.1).

In Crane's activity, students share childhood experiences with one another in dyads or small groups. This assessment could be further adapted to include student encounters with drama, art, poetry, or photography.

Meditation and relaxation exercises can be useful in preparing students for class. A group mandala can be made during the first class meeting in order to build trust between students (Ziff & Beamish, 2004). These relaxing activities send a message that the classroom space, peer interactions, and the learning process are special and sacred.

Main Activities

Expressive arts and play therapy activities described in the previous chapters of this book can serve as main activities during instruction. Engagement in these activities will motivate students to try them with clients. The following activities are specific to classroom instruction.

Creative Concepts

In order to help students increase their comprehension of classroom concepts, students can draw an assigned concept while other students guess what it is (Guevara, 2002). Alternatively, students can create a concept map to illustrate the relationship between clients, therapists, toys, art, play, creativity, and healing. Students might also use psychodrama, poetry, music, or sandplay figurines to symbolically communicate concepts.

Figure 10.2 is an example of a sandplay therapy scene based on the prompt, "What does expressive arts mean to me?" Students were asked to bring a tin aluminum pan and uncooked rice to class for their sandtray.

Jigsaw Puzzle

In the group activity of jigsaw puzzle, students are assigned to four or more colored teams, such as red, blue, green, and purple (Bonwell & Eison, 1991). Within the colored teams, the students are given a number

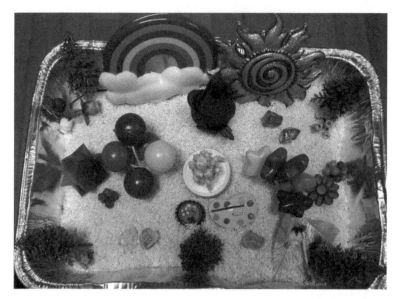

Figure 10.2   What Does Expressive Arts Mean to Me?

from one to four. Then students go to their numbered groups to discuss and become an expert on their assigned concept(s). For example, the instructor may assign group one Axline's basic principles 1 and 2, group two Axline's basic principles 3 and 4, and so on. After 10 minutes of discussion, group members go back to their colored teams (red, blue, green, etc.) to explain their assigned concept to the rest of the group. Students in group number one begin first. This activity allows each student to become an expert on one concept. For added creativity, students could incorporate art or psychodrama to act out their concept.

Role-Play

Although role-play is a common activity in classrooms, many students may feel awkward, especially when students playing the role of clients are not convincing. Novice students may disclose too much about themselves as clients or may unknowingly help the students playing the role of the therapist. Some students may also feel uncomfortable knowing such personal information about fellow classmates (Smith, 2009; Werner-Wilson, 2001).

Several authors (Ballon et al., 2007; Dunn-Snow & Joy-Smellie, 2000; Vernon & Tollerud, 2001) provide helpful ideas for addressing these concerns. They recommend beginning with nontherapeutic role-play scenarios. For role-plays performed in front of the entire group of students, instructors should choose willing participants or those who seem the least shy to serve as therapist and client. It is important to remind students that they can stop at any time. Students who are observing can be engaged by writing down positive and constructive feedback to share later either orally or in writing. Students are encouraged to give the "gift of honest feedback" (Larson, 2004, p. 17). When debriefing, instructors ask the students in the roles of therapist and client what they were feeling during particular times of the session.

Werner-Wilson (2001) suggests that instructors find theatre students to serve as clients. The theatre students can provide feedback to the students in the role of therapist, while theatre faculty deliver feedback to the theatre students on their acting skills. The instructor may also choose to be the client, or a student may play the role of a fictional character as the client (Smith, 2009; Woodward, 1999). Students might create a fictional client by inventing a name, demographic information, presenting problem, triggering event, and conscious and unconscious client desires (Shepard, 2002, as cited in Smith, 2009).

Closure Activities

Closure activities provide a ritual ending that signals a time to prepare to transition to another environment. One creative closing exercise involves students reflecting on what is most important in their learning (Warren et al., 2012). They summarize and integrate what they have learned by making a bookmark, index card, or poster with the information. Deaver and Shiflett (2011) recommend that students artistically represent important concepts through drawing or collage.

With advanced students or those nearing the end of a course in expressive arts or play therapy, the first author (Crane) asks students to create a picture that shows what they believe about the therapeutic process. After creating their *This I Believe* picture, students share and process the pictures with one another. Students tend to either apply a metaphor to therapy or use images and words to convey meaning, as seen in Figure 10.3. This activity is based on the National Public Radio Series, *This I Believe*, and the series of books by the same name (Allison & Gediman, 2007).

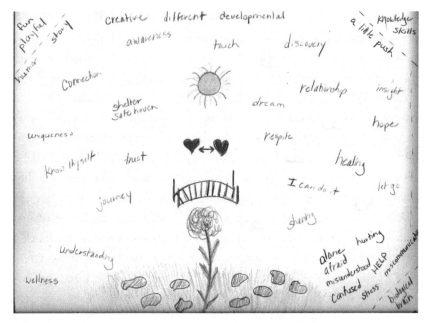

Figure 10.3   This I Beleive

Instructor Involvement

Instructors may wonder what to do while the students are engaged in an activity. They can participate along with the students, which can help the students not feel watched. However, instructors need to monitor how much they reveal of themselves. A helpful suggestion is for instructors to create something that references the group process and gives students immediate feedback (Boldt & Paul, 2011). For instance, if the instructor witnesses students discussing topics that are unrelated to class, he or she might symbolically represent this observation by drawing a soccer ball rolling down a hill away from the children on the soccer field.

One additional difficulty is that instructors must learn to work within their given amount of class time (Guevara, 2002). It is possible that an overly enthusiastic instructor may focus too much on activities as a way to make students feel good or to flaunt their "bag of tricks" (Guevara, 2002). Although instructors should be prepared for class time, overplanning can interfere with the need for flexibility and flow during the class session. Class time should reflect a fluctuating process of engagement and learning through brief 12-minute lectures and then activities, reflection, and application to their personal and professional experiences outside of the classroom (Boldt & Paul, 2011; Grainer et al., 2004; Guevara, 2002).

CEL CLASSROOM SCENARIO

In a family play therapy workshop, the second author (Baggerly) taught students how to lead clients in the *Kinetic Family Drawing*. She provided informed consent and invited students to participate at an emotional level of challenge but not overwhelming frustration. The instructor reminded the group, "Together we create an atmosphere of warmth and nonjudgmental acceptance." As a warm-up activity, the instructor asked students to form small groups to share or describe a favorite family photo from their childhood. Students were to name who was in the photo and three characteristics of each family member.

For the main activity, the instructor asked students to remember their family structure when they were 8 to 10 years old. They were given 15 minutes to do their Kinetic Family Drawing of their childhood family. They were asked to draw on a paper each family member doing something. The instructor dimmed the florescent lights to emphasize natural lights and played soft meditative music on the computer. The instructor informed students when they had five minutes left for their drawing.

For a transition, the instructor turned off the music. She asked students to get into groups of three or four to share their drawings. A list of questions was provided to the groups, so members could help the drawers process their pictures. For example, "What was this person thinking and feeling?", "What are your thoughts and feelings about the distance between this one and that one?", "What does this one need?", "What do you wish the family was doing together?", and "How might this impact your therapy with future clients?"

One student shared her drawing of sitting in a car with her father, stepmother, and stepsister and waving good-bye to her mother, who was crying on the front porch of her house. She stated that this was her experience every other weekend. When her classmates asked what the little girl (the student) was feeling in the picture, she said, "Happy that I was with my stepsister but guilty that my mother was crying." The student began to cry and express her grief and frustration of having to carry such a heavy burden as a child. When asked what this little girl (the student) needs, she said, "For my mother to smile and say, 'Have fun, and I'll be happy to hear all about it when you get back.'" The instructor walked by and asked the student to give this gift of permission to herself. The student indicated that she needed time to quietly reflect on what this would mean for her.

To utilize the strength and comfort of the small group, the instructor asked other members if any of them felt such a heavy burden for their parent, and how/if they gave themselves permission to have fun. Other members shared common experiences of parent illnesses and family poverty. Yet, later they permitted themselves the freedom to enjoy hot baths and spending sprees. Hearing other group members' experiences provided the student with enough time and space to process internally.

During the large group closure activity, the instructor asked for volunteers to share insights they experienced. The aforementioned student shared that her Kinetic Family Drawing helped her realize that she spends so much time protecting her daughter from separation anxiety and that she rarely gives herself permission to enjoy alone time with her husband. She committed that she would give herself the gift of enjoying a weekend alone with her husband once a month. When prompted to share how this activity may impact her clients, the student stated that prior to the activity, she was inclined to shield herself and children from acknowledging their deep grief. However, now she stated that she would give children the freedom to experience their grief while preserving the joy of childhood.

CONCLUSION

Creative experiential learning can be the pedagogy of the optimistic play and art therapist. CEL allows students to engage in activities, reflect, discover connections, make new meaning, and apply learning. Benefits of this social constructionist educational method are increased self-expression, openness, self-awareness, self-acceptance, empathy, problem solving, self-care, and direct experiential knowledge.

Instructor preparation entails developing general pedagogical skills, such as creating a positive and trusting environment, engaging students, facilitating discussions, pacing, managing conflict, and maintaining ethical principles and boundaries. Physical preparation includes preparing enough space and materials. Student preparation occurs by encouraging students to take ownership of their learning, addressing initial resistance, normalizing vulnerability, and varying group size.

The process of CEL involves informed consent, formative assessment, variation of method and media, continual encouragement, and processing and debriefing. Instructors lead students in warm-up activities, main activities, and closure activities to facilitate learning. When instructors implement CEL to teach expressive arts and play therapy, they enrich the lives of students, children, and society. CEL is the pedagogy of the optimistic play and art therapist.

REFERENCES

Allison, J., & Gediman, D. (Eds.). (2007). *This I believe: The personal philosophies of remarkable men and women.* New York, NY: Holt.

Axline, V. M. (1947). *Play therapy.* New York, NY: Ballantine Books.

Baggerly, J. N. (2002). Practical technological applications to promote pedagogical principles and active learning in counselor education. *Journal of Technology in Counseling, 2*(2). Retrieved from http://jtc.col state.edu/vol2_2/index.htm

Ballon, B. C., Silver, I., & Fidler, D. (2007). Headspace theatre: An innovative method for experiential learning of psychiatric symptomatology using modified role-playing and improvisational theatre techniques. *Academic Psychiatry, 31*(5), 380–387.

Beck, M. (1999). *Expecting Adam: A true story of birth, rebirth, and everyday magic.* New York, NY: Berkley.

Bleakley, A. (2004). "Your creativity or mine?" A typology of creativities in higher education and the value of a pluralistic approach. *Teaching in Higher Education, 9*(4), 463–475.

Boldt, R. W., & Paul, S. (2011). Building a creative-arts therapy group at a university counseling center. *Journal of College Student Psychotherapy, 25*(1), 39–52.

Bonwell, C., & Eison, J. (1991). *Active learning: Creating excitement in the classroom.* ERIC Higher Education Report No. 1. Washington, DC: George Washington University.

Brown, B. (2010). *The gifts of imperfection: Let go of who you think you're supposed to be and embrace who you are.* Center City, MN: Hazelden.

Center for Play Therapy (Producer). (1994). *Cookies, choices & kids: A creative approach to discipline* [DVD]. Denton, TX: Author.

Clegg, P. (2008). Creativity and critical thinking in the globalised university. *Innovations in Education & Teaching International, 45*(3), 219–226.

Dale, E. (1969). *Audio-visual methods in teaching.* New York, NY: Holt, Rinehart, & Winston.

Deaver, S. P., & Shiflett, C. (2011). Art-based supervision techniques. *The Clinical Supervisor, 30*(2), 257–276.

Detorie, R. *One big happy* [Cartoon]. Creators Syndicate.

Dunn-Snow, P., & Joy-Smellie, S. (2000). Teaching art therapy techniques: Mask-making, a case in point. *Art therapy: Journal of the American Art Therapy Association, 17*(2), 125–131.

Edelson, P. J. (1999). Creativity and adult education. *New Directions for Adult & Continuing Education, 81,* 3–13.

Gibson, R. (2010). The "art" of creative teaching: Implications for higher education. *Teaching in Higher Education, 15*(5), 607–613.

Grainer, T., Barnes, J., & Scoffham, S. (2004). A creative cocktail: Creative teaching in initial teacher education. *Journal of Education for Teaching, 30*(3), 243–253.

Guevara, J. R. (2002). More than a "bag of tricks": Using creative methodologies in environmental adult and community education. *Adult Learning, 13*(2), 24–29.

Hargreaves, J. (2008). Risk: The ethics of a creative curriculum. *Innovations in Education & Teaching International, 45*(3), 227–234.

Henshon, S. E. (2009). Highly inventive explorer of creativity: An interview with John Baer. *Roeper Review, 31*(1), 3–7.

Johnson, C. (1955). *Harold and the purple crayon.* New York, NY: Harper Collins.

Johnson, L. *For better or for worse* [Cartoon]. United Feature Syndicate.

Jones, A. T. (1992). Mask making: The use of the expressive arts in leadership development. *Journal of Experiential Education, 15*(1), 28–34.

Keane, B., & Keane, J. *The family circus* [Cartoon]. King Features Syndicate.

Kleiman, P. (2008). Towards transformation: Conceptions of creativity in higher education. *Innovations in Education and Teaching International, 45*(3), 209–217.

Larson, R. T. (2004). Training in the teaching arts: A case study from the Paul A. Kaplan Center for Educational Drama. *Teaching Artist Journal, 2*(1), 12–19.

Livingston, L. (2010). Teaching creativity in higher education. *Arts Education Policy Review, 111*(2), 59–62.

Malchiodi, C. A. (2007). *The art therapy sourcebook.* New York, NY: McGraw-Hill.

McCauliffe, G., & Eriksen, K. (Eds.). (2011). *Handbook of counselor preparation: Constructivist, developmental, and experiential approaches.* Los Angeles, CA: Sage.

Ogunleye, J. (2002). Creative approaches to raising achievement of adult learners in English further education. *Journal of Further & Higher Education, 26*(2), 173–181.

Portis, A. (2006). *Not a box.* New York, NY: HarperCollins.

Portis, A. (2008). *Not a stick.* New York, NY: HarperCollins.

Reynolds, P. H. (2003). *The dot.* Cambridge, MA: Candlewick.

Reynolds, P. H. (2004). *Ish.* Cambridge, MA: Candlewick.

Rogers, F. (2003). *The world according to Mister Rogers: Important things to remember.* New York, NY: Hyperion.

Rogers, F. (2006). *Many ways to say I love you: Wisdom for parents and children from Mister Rogers.* New York, NY: Hyperion.

Saltzberg, B. (2010). *Beautiful oops!* New York, NY: Workman.

Schulz, C. M. *Peanuts* [Cartoon]. United Feature Syndicate.

Smith, A. L. (2009). Role play in counselor education and supervision: Innovative ideas, gaps, and future directions. *Journal of Creativity in Mental Health, 4*(2), 124–138.

Sori, C. F. (2003). Therapist attitudes about play. In C. F. Sori & L. L. Hecker (Eds.), *The therapist's notebook for children and adolescents: Homework, handouts, and activities for use in psychotherapy* (pp. xxvii–xxix). Binghamton, NY: Haworth.

Vernon, A., & Tollerud, T. R. (2001). Transformative learning experiences in graduate classes on counseling children and adolescents. In K. Eriksen & G. McAuliffe (Eds.), *Teaching counselors and therapists: Constructivist and developmental course design* (pp. 219–233). Westport, CT: Bergin & Garvey.

Warren, J., Zavaschi, G., Covello, C., & Zakaria, N. S. (2012). The use of bookmarks in teaching counseling ethics. *Journal of Creativity in Mental Health, 7*(2), 187–201.

Watterson, B. *Calvin & Hobbes* [Cartoon]. Universal Press Syndicate.

Werner-Wilson, R. J. (2001). Experiential exercises in MFT training: Gender, power, and diversity. *Contemporary Family Therapy: An International Journal, 23*(2), 221–229.

Woodward, A. L. (1999). Infants' ability to distinguish between purposeful and non-purposeful behaviors. *Infant Behavior and Development, 22*, 145–160.

Ziff, K. K., & Beamish, P. M. (2004). Teaching a course on the arts and counseling: Experiential learning in counselor education. *Counselor Education & Supervision, 44*(2), 147–159.

11

Integrating Play and Expressive Art Therapy Into Small Group Counseling With Preadolescents: A Humanistic Approach

SUE C. BRATTON, DALENA DILLMAN TAYLOR, AND SINEM AKAY

INTRODUCTION

In art or play the child may do the impossible. He or she may fulfill symbolically both positive wishes and negative impulses, without fear of real consequences. He or she can learn to control the real world by experimenting with active mastery of tools, media, and the ideas and feelings expressed in the process. He or she can gain symbolic access to and relive past traumas, and can rehearse and practice for the future. He or she can learn to be in charge in a symbolic mode, and thus come to feel competent to master reality. (Rubin, 1984, p. 29)

The importance of play and art in children's lives is widely acknowledged by experts in the fields of child development, child mental health, and neurobiology (Badenoch, 2008; Brown, 2009; Gil, 2010; Landreth, 2012; Malchiodi, 2008; Oaklander, 2007; Panksepp, 2004; Perry, 2006; Rubin, 2005; Schaefer, 2011). Although established as distinct therapeutic modalities with specific education, training, and supervision requirements, play therapy (Association for Play Therapy [APT], 2013) and expressive/creative arts therapies (National Coalition of Creative Arts Therapies Associations [NCCATA], 2013; International Expressive Arts Therapy Association [IEATA], 2013) were founded on similar beliefs in the therapeutic properties of play and art media as nonthreatening and symbolic means of expression.

As early as the 1920s, child therapists provided play materials for children to express themselves and to facilitate the healing process. Today, play therapy is widely accepted as a developmentally responsive mental health intervention for children (Landreth, 2012; Schaefer, 2011) with a substantial and growing base of research to support its effectiveness with various presenting issues and populations (Baggerly, Ray, & Bratton, 2010; Bratton, Ray, Rhine, & Jones, 2005; Reddy, Files-Hall, & Schaefer, 2005). Although the therapeutic needs of preadolescent children received attention in the play therapy literature in the 1940s through the 1970s (Ginott, 1961; Schiffer, 1952; Slavson & Redl, 1944; Slavson & Schiffer, 1975), the vast majority of literature and research since the 1940s is focused on play therapy's use and effectiveness with children under 10 years of age (Center for Play Therapy, 2013).

The use of art as a therapeutic modality with children emerged in the 1940s (Rubin, 2010), although research evidence is in its infancy (Kapitan, 2010). The use of the terms *expressive* and *creative arts* to reflect broader therapeutic modalities that include art, drama, movement/dance, poetry/writing, and other creative processes (IEAT, 2013; NCCATA, 2013) emerged in the latter half of the 20th century. Proponents of these modalities advocated the use of a variety of expressive mediums in their work with older children, who naturally use art and symbols to express themselves (Chapman, 1993; Gil, 1991, 2010; Landgarten, 1981; Malchiodi, 2005; Oaklander, 1988, 2007; Rubin, 2005). A review of contemporary literature revealed a handful of outcome studies examining the effect of art therapy modalities for children (Chapman, Morabito, Ladakakos, Schreier, & Knudson, 2001; Favara-Scacco, Smirne, Schiliro, & Di Cataldo, 2001; Lyshak-Stelzer, Singer,

St. John, & Chemtob, 2007; Pifalo, 2002, 2006; Smitheman-Brown & Church, 1996). Study findings were promising, but overall the results were limited by small sample sizes and lack of control groups.

Over the past 10 years, researchers in the field of play therapy demonstrated a renewed interest in interventions targeting preadolescent children. Findings from five randomized, controlled studies suggested that integrating expressive arts and group play therapy within a humanistic framework was an effective and developmentally and culturally responsive treatment modality for children in this phase of development (Flahive & Ray, 2007; Ojiambo & Bratton, in press; Packman & Bratton, 2003; Shen, 2007; Shen & Armstrong, 2008).

This chapter provides an overview of developmental, theoretical, and therapeutic rationales for integrating group play therapy and expressive arts for troubled preadolescents. As individual modalities, play therapy and the various expressive art therapies are described in detail elsewhere in this book, along with criteria for ethical practice. We describe the process and procedures for implementing an integrated play therapy–expressive arts model and conclude with a case example to illustrate the therapeutic process and to provide practical examples of expressive activities that play therapists with training and experience in the use of expressive media can incorporate into their current work. As authors, we want to be transparent that our primary training and experience is play therapy. We do not hold any certification in the fields of expressive, creative, or art therapy. The first author is a Registered Play Therapist and Supervisor (RPT-S) with more than 20 years of experience using play therapy, group play therapy, and expressive/creative arts from a humanistic theoretical orientation. As with any mental health intervention, ethical practice requires clinicians to (a) obtain training in the specified treatment modality—in this case, play therapy, expressive arts, and group processes specific to this age group—and (b) exercise clinical judgment in determining client appropriateness for the treatment and specific techniques or activities presented.

Play Therapy With Preadolescents

Preadolescence, defined as a period of development encompassing the ages of approximately 9 to 13 years (Bratton, Ceballos, & Ferebee, 2009; Oesterreich, 1995), is a period of rapid change for children. Children in this developmental phase are shifting from concrete thinking that is externalized primarily through their play to an emerging capacity for internal processes and abstract thought that is not fully developed until around 15 years of age (Piaget, 1977; Vygotsky, 1966). Similar to the developmental rationale for play therapy with younger children, play, activity, and art provide preadolescents with a developmentally responsive means to bridge the gap between concrete and abstract thought processes (Ginott, 1994; Landreth, 2012). Yet, their play preferences and needs are different and require play therapists who work with this age group to purposefully select materials and activities to optimally facilitate their growth and healing.

During this phase of development, peers hold tremendous importance. Children begin to shift from dependence on parents to increased need for peer relationships (Akos & Martin, 2003; Hamachek, 1988). Erikson (1980) characterized this phase in children's social development as industry versus inferiority, a time in which preadolescents strive to be competent and productive and value social interaction and connection with peers. The desire to find a sense of belonging with peers serves as motivation to modify behavior for acceptance (Ginott, 1994) and can be used to therapeutic advantage.

From a developmental perspective and when clinically indicated, group interventions offer potential therapeutic benefit for preteens over individual treatment formats (Akos, Hamm, Mack, & Dunaway, 2007; Armstrong, 2008; Draper, Ritter, & Willingham, 2003; Gerrity & DeLucia-Waack, 2007). Although research and literature on the process and effects of group play therapy with preadolescent children is scarce (Bratton & Ferebee, 1999; Ojiambo & Bratton, in press; Packman & Bratton, 2003), several play therapy authors described its therapeutic advantages, as well as potential challenges (Bratton et al., 2009; Ginott, 1961, 1994; Landreth, 2012; Ray, 2011; Slavson & Schiffer, 1975; Sweeney & Homeyer, 1999).

Expressive Arts Therapy

Rogers (1993) stated that part of the therapeutic process is to awaken creative capacity. According to IEAT (2013), "integrating the arts processes and allowing one to flow into another permits individuals to access inner resources for healing, clarity, illumination and creativity." The expressive and creative arts include such things as drawing, painting, sculpting, music, movement, writing, phototherapy, collage, sandplay, imagery, fantasy, drama, improvisation, puppetry, and woodworking. For preadolescents who are naturally concerned about others' evaluation, art media provides a symbolic and nonthreatening means of self-expression. Through the various expressive art forms, preteens can engage in a creative process that promotes an understanding of self and other and a sense of competence and mastery—important developmental tasks for this age group.

Malchiodi (2005) emphasized the value of self-selected expressive arts activities to facilitate a creative process of self-exploration that connects mind and body; a process that stimulates all of the senses (e.g., sight, touch, taste, smell, and hearing) and enables access to the right hemisphere of the brain (Badenoch, 2008). The use of expressive media offers preadolescents greater access to experiences, thoughts, and feelings that might not otherwise be explored or noticed, thus enhancing the connections between left and right brain that are necessary for integration and healing (Badenoch, 2008). Furthermore, the self-creative process awakened during therapy serves as a protective factor by providing preadolescents with an internal structure for coping with future challenges (Rubin, 2005).

INTEGRATING PLAY AND EXPRESSIVE ART THERAPY INTO SMALL GROUP COUNSELING WITH PREADOLESCENTS: PROCESS AND PROCEDURES

Integrating expressive arts and humanistic play therapy principles and procedures within a small group format offers preadolescent children a developmentally responsive and effective means to freely explore their thoughts and feelings, and further provides unique opportunities to examine their perceptions about self and others. We provide an overview of the model including theoretical framework and describe the format and structure, materials and space needs, considerations for the use of therapist-offered expressive art activities, and a brief summary of research supporting the modality.

Humanistic Theoretical Framework

This integrated group play therapy–expressive arts model is grounded in humanistic principles and procedures. Early proponents of group play therapy with preadolescents espoused a nondirective approach based on a belief that older children benefited from the opportunity to express themselves and direct their own activitiy (Schiffer, 1952; Slavson & Redl, 1944). According to Malchiodi (2005) and Rogers (1993), expressive/creative therapies are well-suited to a humanistic approach. A humanistic approach requires a profound trust in the individual's innate capacity for self-direction and to make choices that are self-enhancing. Bratton and Ray (2002) defined humanistic play therapy as belief in (a) the child's natural striving toward growth, mastery, and maturity; (b) the child's capacity for self-direction, self-regulation, self-responsibility, and socialization; and (c) the essential nature of the therapeutic relationship in facilitating the child's growth. Foundational to this approach is the belief that spontaneous and self-directed play and creative expression, within an unconditional and trusting relationship, is the primary source of intra- and interpersonal growth and lasting change. According to Rubin (1984), "child[ren] cannot learn to control and organize [the] self, if the structure does not ultimately come from within" (p. 29).

From a humanistic stance, the play therapist's first objective is to create a therapeutic space for healing and growth. Because of the importance that preadolescents place on peers' opinions, they are often self-conscious and hesitant to engage with other group members in the initial phase of therapy. Therapist-guided activities can reduce group members' anxiety and establish a sense of comfort by providing a structure that facilitates a safe experience in which group members can non-verbally and verbally interact and connect. Davis (2002) underscored the value of structuring expressive art activities within a person-centered approach as a means of facilitating psychological contact. Bratton et al. (2009) discussed additional benefits of therapist-offered art experiences, including introducing preadolescents to an expressive art form with which they may be unfamiliar or hesitant to try on their own, and later in the therapeutic process, creating experiences that encourage collaboration and problem solving.

Wilson and Ryan (2005) emphasized that from a nondirective perspective therapist-presented activities are used in response to preadolescent children's needs and immediate experience in play therapy as opposed to planned, directive techniques. Ojiambo and Bratton (in press) supported this view and added that the humanistic play therapist's intent is never to direct the individual or group process toward the completion of a product, but rather the objective is to offer opportunities for, and serve as a witness to, creative expression that fosters group members' greater understanding of self and other.

Structure and Format

Historically, there have been two main schools of thought regarding the therapist's role and use of art media in expressive therapies (Rubin, 1984) and group play approaches with preadolescents (Bratton & Ferebee, 1999): unstructured and structured. Gil (2006) suggested that many play therapists rigidly adhere to a nondirective or directive approach, and instead recommended a more integrative approach to best meet clients' needs. Rubin made a clear distinction between the use of structured and unstructured art experiences with groups and discussed the advantages and limitations of each.

We prescribe to a model in which the play therapist flexibly responds to group members' needs by providing ample opportunities for unstructured play along with creating, as determined necessary, therapist-guided experiences with expressive media. The balance between use of semistructured and unstructured play and activities is based on the clinician's understanding of the unique needs of group members, the stage of group development, and the therapist's theoretical guide. From a humanistic perspective, overstructuring of groups inhibits growth. As noted previously, expressive art activities are offered to reduce anxiety, establish a sense of safety, foster connection and interaction among group members, and, as group members become more comfortable with each other, to provide opportunities to draw on internal resources and experiment with more self-enhancing and satisfying ways of relating to each other. The intent is to facilitate a creative process that becomes increasingly self- and group-directed and permits preadolescents to draw on and develop their internal resources as they explore, create, negotiate, problem solve, and resolve conflicts that naturally emerge in an unstructured process.

Ojiambo and Bratton (in press) provided a protocol for integrating expressive arts and group play therapy within a humanistic format. Although the structure and format can vary depending on the needs of group members and the setting, the authors proposed a structure for a school-based, 16-session protocol that included opportunities for self-directed and group-directed activities as well as semi-structured activities offered by the therapist as needed. The protocol specified weekly 50-minute sessions and a group size of three preadolescents to allow sufficient time for creating and processing. Roughly 10 minutes at the end of each session was allocated for closure and sharing among group members to facilitate transition back to the classroom. In the initial sessions, the structure consisted of approximately 20 minutes of a therapist-offered expressive art experience followed by 20 minutes of self-directed play/activity. The authors found that as preadolescents felt safe in the group, they naturally assumed more responsibility and self-direction and required less structure from the play therapist.

Although the model utilizes a small group format based on a developmental rationale for enhancing therapeutic benefit, there are instances when group play therapy is counter-indicated. A discussion on selection of group members is beyond the scope of this chapter, but Bratton et al. (2009) and Ginott (1994) discussed selection criteria for preadolescent groups and provided guidelines for screening group members.

Space and Materials

Preteens are highly active and have varied interests. Play therapists purposefully plan the space and materials with their developmental needs in mind. A space of approximately 200 square feet is minimally sufficient to allow for group and individual work space for a group of up to four preadolescents. Inadequate space increases the potential for frustration and conflict among group members. In minimal spaces, moveable furniture and equipment permits the therapist and group members to move furniture to create space as needed. In our experience, preadolescents enjoy the freedom to rearrange the room to create their own space. Equipment and materials are selected to reflect group members' cultural experiences and to stimulate group interaction, promote creative self-expression, encourage exploration and release of feelings, facilitate acting out of real-life experiences or concerns, and encourage problem solving, negotiating, and coping strategies. Bratton and Ferebee (1999) provided a detailed list of furniture, equipment, toys, materials, and expressive media for fully equipping a group play/activity therapy room for this age group. The authors also provided suggestions for accommodating less-than-ideal spaces and restricted budgets.

Expressive Arts Media and Activities

A wide variety of expressive media must be on hand at all times to encourage preadolescents' spontaneous creations using materials that they find most inviting. Materials must be plentiful to accommodate the needs of all group members. For therapist-offered activities, the primary consideration is the perceived level of safety among group members. The humanistic play therapist is flexible and spontaneous in suggesting activities based on the immediate needs and desires of the group; group members are free to participate or not participate, to use materials in their own way, and to change the course and process of an activity at any time (Ojiambo & Bratton, in press). The focus is on the creative process within and among group members, with the therapist serving as a non-judgmental witness, yet also responsible for maintaining a space of safety and acceptance of individual expression.

Regardless of theoretical approach, when selecting an expressive art medium for a therapist-guided activity, play therapists must consider each member's emotional readiness and the potential effect of selected expressive media on each child. Landgarten (1987) emphasized the potency of expressive media, stating "it can heighten or lower the client's affective state, influence freedom of self-expression, and circumvent defenses" (p. 7). Expressive mediums impact individuals differently and potentially elicit latent thoughts and feelings that preadolescents might not be ready to address within the group context. For these reasons, therapists' training, supervision, and personal experience with a wide array of expressive material and activities are essential and heightens their sensitivity to the materials and to the process. To assist clinicians in considering the potential impact of media on their clients,

Landgarten developed a chart that listed art mediums on a 10-point continuum from more fluid and difficult to control (wet clay) to more resistant and easier to control (lead pencils) to depict the relationship among art mediums and clients' level of control over their creations.

Based on Landgarten's (1987) chart, and adapted from Bratton et al. (2009), we propose the following framework as a guide to selecting materials and activities for preadolescent groups. In general, the higher the expressive medium is on the chart, the greater sense of control the preadolescent experiences, including control over emotions and thoughts that are out of awareness.

Most Control
Lead pencils
Thin markers
Miniature figures
Dry sand and miniatures
Crayons
Collage materials
Puppets/drama
Model magic/modeling clay
Watercolors/chalk pastels
Wet clay
Least Control

Additional factors influence the degree of control experienced and the impact of the media on the preadolescent: (a) therapist directive for the activity, including the amount of structure presented and the degree to which the activity is related to client issues, (b) therapist processing of activity, such as asking direct questions and linking the creation to client concerns and experiences, (c) combining media in an activity, and (d) group dynamics. For example, in general, we agree with Landgarten (1987) that collage activities in which clients cut and paste images from magazines or similar materials falls in the middle of the art media continuum. However, as we demonstrate in the case example, when collage incorporates multiple media within the concept of mandala-making, the experience can easily elicit deep feelings and thoughts, and thus would move into the lower third of the chart. We encourage clinicians to adapt the chart to fit their experiences, the expressive mediums they use, and their understanding of clients' needs and preferences.

Finally, regardless of theoretical orientation, the play therapist must exercise clinical judgment in determining preadolescents' psychological readiness to engage in sharing and processing personal creations and consider developmental factors, including capacity for abstract thought. From a humanistic approach, preadolescents' experience within the creative process is more important than the activity or resulting product. The therapist consistently conveys attitudes of empathic understanding, unconditional acceptance, and congruence, along with a belief in each group member's capacity for self-regulation, self-responsibility, and socialization. Bratton et al. (2009) offered additional guidelines and examples for processing expressive arts activities within a humanistic framework.

Research Support

Numerous controlled-outcome studies demonstrate the effectiveness of humanistic play therapy interventions with children under 10 years old (Baggerly et al., 2010; Bratton et al., 2005). A review of literature revealed a scarcity of play therapy outcome research targeting older children and even less focused on the incorporation of expressive arts activities into play therapy. Of the handful of experimental studies examining the effects of play therapy interventions using expressive arts (Flahive & Ray, 2007; Ojiambo & Bratton, in press; Packman & Bratton, 2003; Shen, 2007; Shen & Armstrong, 2008), all five studies followed humanistic principles, used a small group format, were conducted in school settings over the past decade, and reported statistically significant beneficial outcomes and moderate to large treatment effects. The three studies that were most similar to the presented model are reviewed as follows. We omitted studies that limited the intervention to a single expressive art medium. In the studies eliminated, only sandtray and miniatures were used (Flahive & Ray; Shen & Armstrong).

In a randomized, controlled study, Packman and Bratton (2003) examined the effects of using expressive art activities (e.g., collage, drawing, clay, sandtray, and puppetry) within a humanistic group play therapy format with 29 preadolescents, 10 to 12 years of age, who were diagnosed with learning difficulties. According to parent report, the experimental group ($n = 15$) demonstrated statistically significant reductions ($p < .05$) and large treatment effects on total behavior problems and internalizing behavior problems compared to the wait-list control group. The group play therapy intervention demonstrated moderate to large treatment effects on externalizing behavior problems, although the results were not statistically significant.

Ojiambo and Bratton (in press) conducted a randomized, controlled study based on the protocol used in Packman and Bratton (2003) and named the treatment model Group Activity Play Therapy (GAPT). The researchers examined the effectiveness of GAPT with 60 displaced Ugandan orphans, aged 10 to 12 years, exhibiting clinical levels of behavior problems. Teachers and housemothers, blinded to participant group assignment, reported that experimental group children demonstrated statistically significant reductions ($p < .025$) in externalizing and internalizing behavior problems compared to the active control (Reading Mentoring), and that GAPT demonstrated moderate to large treatment effects. The results of this study are especially promising because of the consistency of findings from two sources of measurement for each outcome variable and the use of procedures to blind assessors to the study.

Shen (2007) randomly assigned 73 Taiwanese seventh and eighth graders to the Gestalt expressive group play therapy treatment ($n = 24$), a group cognitive-verbal treatment ($n = 25$), or a no-treatment control group ($n = 24$). Results from teacher and parent report were mixed. Teachers reported statistically significant improvement in behavioral and emotional strength for both treatment groups, with the Gestalt expressive arts group intervention making the greatest gains. Parents reported no significant improvement on the same measures. For school and social adjustment, neither treatment group demonstrated significant gains.

PRACTICAL APPLICATION

The following case example demonstrates the integration of expressive art activities and play therapy for preadolescents. The case example is a composite of client features. Identifying information is disguised to protect confidentiality. We present sample activities and procedures within a humanistic group process, but the activities presented are easily adapted for use with individual preadolescents and for use by therapists adhering to other theoretical orientations.

Because of space constraints, we focus greater attention on the use of therapist-offered activities than on group-directed play. To illustrate the therapeutic process, as well as considerations for selecting expressive media (Landgarten, 1987) and processing activities, we selected three examples of semistructured activities from the beginning, middle, and end of the play therapy process. See Bratton and Ferebee (1999) for further examples of expressive activities for use with preadolescent groups. Other resources for expressive/creative activities that can be adapted for children in this age group include Oaklander (1988) and Malchiodi (2002). Bratton and Ferebee (1999) also provided descriptions of equipment, toys, and materials for a fully equipped activity/playroom for preadolescents, similar to the playroom used in the case example. Although we suggest specific activities in this section, from a humanistic perspective group members are free to creatively interpret and modify activities according to their needs. The play therapist exercises clinical judgment in sharing observations of group members' creative process, and although preadolescents are invited to verbally share their creations with each other, the therapist maintains an attitude of respect and acceptance of group members' right to choose not to participate. At all times, the play therapist is flexible and responsive to the immediate needs and preferences of group members. The format and structure for this group followed the Ojiambo and Bratton (in press) protocol previously described.

Case Study

Monique, Isabelle, and Beatrice were 12 years old at the time of referral. They were referred by their fifth-grade teachers for emotional and behavioral concerns related to excessive perfectionism that interfered with their academic performance. They were screened prior to selection to the group (Bratton et al., 2009). Exclusion criteria included significant developmental delays, history of interpersonal trauma, and inability to connect with others.

Per teacher report, Monique demonstrated aggressive behaviors in the classroom when she felt criticized by her peers or teacher and refused to take math tests because of a fear of failure. Monique demonstrated leadership potential, but at times her peers viewed her as bossy and overwhelming. Monique lived with her biological mother, stepdad of two years, 14-year-old sister, and 7-year-old brother. Monique's mother described her as a good girl and reported no concerns regarding her behavior.

Isabelle's teacher described her as gifted but extremely withdrawn, and further noted that Isabelle refused to participate in class discussions or group projects. Isabelle lived with her mother, a professional who traveled frequently, and her 18-year-old sister, who cared for Isabelle when her mother was away from home. Isabelle's mother consented for her to participate in counseling but failed to return any phone calls.

According to Beatrice's teacher, she demonstrated excessive anxiety related to test-taking and failed to complete time-limited tasks because of incessant corrections. In group projects, she showed no difficulty. Beatrice had many friends, although she tended to go along with what others suggested. Beatrice's parents reported that she was obsessed with her weight and appearance, despite recent weight loss, and constantly compared herself to her sister. They expressed concern that Beatrice was developing an eating disorder. Beatrice lived with her biological parents and 15-year-old sister, who participated in the gifted program at her school.

Monique, Isabelle, and Beatrice participated in group play therapy one time per week for 50 minutes at the elementary school they attended. The group met a total of 15 weeks in the fall semester. Sessions were held whether or not all members were present. A variety of expressive art activities were offered by the play therapist over the course of therapy. In the following examples, the therapist carefully considered group members' emotional readiness, the perceived level of safety in the group, and group members' presenting issues related to perfectionism in selecting expressive media and activities. Because of space constraints, only portions of each activity and group members' creations are described.

Beginning Phase: Sandtray and Miniature Figures

Sandplay therapists (De Domenico, 1999; Kalff, 1971; Kestly, 2010; Lowenfeld, 1979) advocated the therapeutic use of sand and miniatures with children. Kestly explicitly recommended the modality for preadolescents as an inviting medium "to explore the world that lies between childhood and adulthood" (p. 19). Draper et al. (2003) suggested the use of sand and miniatures to create a safe, nonthreatening environment to help preteens get acquainted and work on their social skills and interpersonal difficulties.

A wide assortment of miniature figures offers preadolescents the opportunity for meaningful self-expression through the safety of symbols, with a moderate level of control over the creative experience, and without worry regarding artistic ability. Although similar activities using miniatures can be presented with or without sand, dry sand can have a soothing effect and decrease anxiety. Based on Landgarten's (1987) guide for selecting expressive mediums and our experience with preadolescent groups, wet sand is typically not offered in a therapist-structured activity during the beginning phase of therapy. The introduction to the sandtray experience varies based on the therapist's theoretical orientation, the purpose of the group, and the needs of group members. Homeyer and Sweeney (2010) offered a comprehensive, nontheoretical overview of possible prompts and methods of introducing sandtray appropriate for children in this age group that range along the continuum of nondirective to directive.

In the case example and specific to the girls' shared issue regarding perfectionism, a sandtray activity was presented in session three to reduce their anxiety and self-consciousness, as an alternative to art mediums such as drawing, about which group members had already expressed inhibitions, and most important, to facilitate a nonthreatening means for group members to connect and share their experiences. For groups in which preadolescents have significant trauma histories, the use of sand at this phase of therapy should be carefully considered. In addition, according to Armstrong (2008), therapists must use caution in processing sandtrays with children in this developmental phase. The experience can evoke strong feelings that preadolescents may be unaware of and have difficulty accepting or sharing with others.

Materials Needed

Although there is no standard collection of miniatures, Bratton and Ferebee (1999) suggested miniatures representative of the following categories: people, animals, fantasy figures, buildings, vehicles, structures, natural objects, vegetation, and symbolic objects. Organization of miniatures by categories allows group members to easily find and access objects they want to use in their sandtrays. Space and cost for group sandtray experiences are typical concerns for play therapists. Traditional sandplay therapists are very specific in their requirement for the size and shape of the sandtray (a wooden tray approximately 20 inches by 29 inches by 3 inches), but the associated cost and storage requirements are prohibitive for many play therapists. Clay-colored plastic drip saucers, approximately 18 inches in diameter and painted blue inside, are one example of an affordable and practical solution that is lightweight and stackable for storage. Tools to shape, smooth, and rake the sand are useful, particularly for preadolescents who are reluctant to get their hands dirty or for those who have sensory issues. Homeyer and Sweeney (2010) provided a useful resource for play therapists who are new to the use of this modality, including practical and affordable ideas for sandtrays and miniatures.

Case Study

After providing Monique, Isabelle, and Beatrice each with an 18-inch plant saucer with fine sand, the play therapist presented a brief overview of the activity "as a way of getting to know each other better." Drawing on the activity last week in which the three girls each shared that going to the beach was a favorite summer vacation, the therapist suggested they spend a few moments smoothing and shaping the sand "like you were at the beach." Touching the sand prompted the girls to share memories of time with family at the beach. Although this happening was not related to the activity and the following prompt was unplanned, the therapist followed the group's direction, and after approximately five minutes when the conversation lulled, the therapist suggested that group members look through the miniatures on the wall and choose a figure to represent each person in their beach memory and make a beach scene in their sandtray.

During the process of creating, the therapist noticed such things as the order and difficulty in selecting figures, the process of placing figures in the tray, and the girls' affect related to the process. It was obvious the girls were reflecting on their choices by the amount of time they spent choosing and placing their figures. Evident from her affect, Monique in particular had difficulty making a decision regarding which figures she wanted, with the end result that her tray was overflowing with figures. The therapist also noted that she had quickly buried a playful-looking puppy along one edge of the tray. Although the therapist sensed the importance of Monique's actions, she did not know until several sessions later that Monique's father had died 3 years earlier. Knowing her history would have been a consideration in choosing sandtray in the context of a group experience in the beginning stage of therapy. After approximately 10 minutes, the therapist determined that the girls' scenes were mostly complete and suggested they take a couple more minutes to place their figures.

Next, the therapist invited group members to share their beach scenes. Because the girls had previously discussed their memories of going to the beach, they seemed more comfortable sharing their scenes than is typical at this stage of group development. Monique got everyone's attention by announcing in a loud voice that she should go first because on her vacation "she went to Hawaii and everyone knows Hawaii has the best beaches." Beatrice and Isabelle looked surprised but did not say anything. Monique began by describing the figures she selected for her mother and stepfather, two large giraffes that she placed in the middle of the tray facing each other and touching faces as if they were kissing. "They kiss all the time," she explained. She next described the two figures that she chose to represent herself as a cheerleader and a small dolphin (that was really a shark) and placed them near the edge of the tray where she had buried the puppy earlier. She then took the rake and pushed the sand to make a body of water around where the giraffes were standing. Monique mumbled to herself, "There! They might as well be on an island by themselves. They don't even know I'm around." The therapist was aware that the other girls seemed a bit overwhelmed, but also wanted Monique to feel heard and accepted. "Sometimes, it feels like your mom and dad just don't have enough time for you." Monique nodded and seemed to make a shift in her internal process. She had the dolphin and some of the other figures in the tray swim over to the giraffes. "Yeah, but sometimes they take us neat places like the beach, and we have fun." The shift in Monique's affect allowed Isabelle and

Beatrice to share similar feelings of feeling left out in their families, although for different reasons. The therapist was especially sensitive to the intensity of Monique's experience and reflected group members' shared feelings as a way to help Monique feel that she was not alone in her experience, as well as to begin to forge connections among group members. After a period of unstructured play, the girls shared a snack, which was their weekly ritual for ending sessions and transitioning back to their classrooms.

Middle Phase: Clay/Model Magic Creature

Clay in its various forms provides preadolescents with an experience that is unique from most other art media because of its more intensely tactile nature (Sholt & Gavron, 2006). Oaklander (1988) advocated the use of clay and emphasized that the medium helps preteens connect with their emotions and experiences. Consistent with Landgarten's (1987) continuum of art media, we find the use of Model Magic or Play-Doh affords group members more control over their experience than wet, or natural, clay; thus, these clay-like materials are typically a better choice for the midphase of group play therapy. For children who have difficulty with messiness or sensory issues, Model Magic is particularly appropriate to introduce them to clay materials. The medium allows preadolescents a sense of mastery and control as they shape and reshape the clay according to their creative notions, without an overly tactile experience. In the case example, Model Magic was selected over clay based on an assessment of the group members' psychological readiness and because of one member's strong intolerance for messiness.

Materials Needed

Provide each group member with a fist-size portion of Model Magic, clay, or similar material, depending on the purpose and readiness of members as discussed earlier. Group members need a firm surface for working with the clay, such as a large plastic serving tray, if the room size does not allow for a group-size table, which is often the case. Supply a selection of tools for shaping, including such items as plastic knives, a rubber mallet, a garlic press, a cheese cutter, and special clay tools. When using natural clay, a larger selection of tools is needed, along with a container of water and wet paper towels. For the specific clay activity used in the case example, group members need access to a variety of craft materials, such as colored cellophane and tissue paper, assorted beads, colored feathers, pipe cleaners, construction paper, plastic straws, dried pasta shapes, markers, and scissors to personalize their creature. A selection of CDs for background music is an option that some preadolescent groups enjoy as they engage in the creative process. In the following example, the girls chose to listen to music while they created.

Case Study

The clay animal/creature activity was presented in session eight, approximately midway in the therapeutic process. The play therapist provided a brief introduction to the activity and gave each group member a fist-size portion of Model Magic. Monique suggested they put on some cool music, and the others agreed to her choice. The play therapist suggested the girls experiment with the medium by rolling, squeezing, smashing, poking, and stretching it. None of the girls had experienced the medium previously and were intrigued by its texture. Isabelle, who was typically very quiet, exclaimed with a smile on her face, "This is cool stuff!" Beatrice agreed, and although Monique was initially hesitant to touch the clay, she especially liked smashing and vigorously poking it to the beat of the music. She clearly enjoyed the release of energy the clay afforded, but at the same time, her anxiety was evident. Because Monique seemed to need more time to get comfortable, and because the other group members obviously enjoyed the experience, the therapist followed the needs of the group and allowed more time experimenting with the clay than is typical for this activity.

After about 8 to 10 minutes of experimenting with the clay, the play therapist introduced the idea of creating an animal/creature that could be an animal with which they were familiar or a creature no one had ever seen, or it could be part animal, part creature. Exhibit 11.1 includes the complete description of this activity, including the guided imagery suggested by the therapist. This specific activity was selected with the group members' needs in mind. Although their struggles with perfectionism were evidenced in group by their concern about their artistic ability, and their finished products had lessened over the past few weeks, presenting the image of a creature never before seen was intended to lessen concern over how their creation looked. The therapist observed that the girls were more immersed in the creative process than in any previous session. Isabelle was much more animated than usual, and Monique was more subdued. The girls especially enjoyed using the craft materials to personalize their creature and "create a place for it to rest" (Exhibit 11.1). Because the girls were so absorbed in the creative process, the play therapist waited until there was about 15 minutes left to suggest it was time to add any other touches to their creation, so that group members would have time to share before snack and going back to class.

Exhibit 11.1   Clay Animal Creatures for Preadolescent Groups

---

Clay Animal Creatures
The use of clay can help preadolescents connect with their emotions and experiences (Oaklander, 1988). Bratton and Ferebee (1999) affirmed the value of clay, adding that the medium can help children and adolescents to develop and enhance their sense of self, because it allows them to have a sense of mastery and control. When using clay, preadolescents are in charge of their creations; they can shape and reshape the clay as necessary, giving them the power to change their creation at any moment. Model Magic or Play-Doh instead of natural clay is typically more appropriate for the beginning to middle stage of preadolescent groups to afford group members more control over their emotions and experience.

Materials Needed
Provide each group member with a fist-size portion of Model Magic, clay, or similar material, depending on the purpose and readiness of members. Group members need a firm surface for working with the clay, such as a large plastic serving tray, if the room size does not allow for a group-size table, which is often the case. Supply a selection of tools for shaping, including such items as plastic knives, a rubber mallet, a garlic press, a cheese cutter, and special clay tools. When using natural clay, a larger selection of tools is needed, along with a container of water and wet paper towels. For the specific clay activity used in the case example, group members need access to a variety of craft materials, such as colored cellophane and tissue paper, assorted beads, colored feathers, pipe cleaners, construction paper, plastic straws, dried pasta shapes, markers, and scissors to personalize their creature.

General Directions
Begin by giving each group a portion of the clay/magic model. The suggestions for experimenting with the medium will vary according to group members' readiness and preferences, as well as the type of clay presented. In general, the play therapist encourages preadolescents to become familiar with their clay by touching, pinching, rolling, squeezing, etc. Depending on the group, the therapist may suggest that group members

explore the clay with their eyes open and again with their eyes closed to experience the tactile nature of the clay more fully. The experience of clay media with eyes closed is often more calming and centering. The therapist can suggest that group members share what they notice about the clay, by asking, "How does it feel? Is it cool or warm? Does it feel different with eyes open or closed? Do you like how it feels?" Group members may experience some anxiety at the beginning, thus sensitivity to their experience and allowing sufficient time to explore the material is important. Having background music is an option that some preadolescent groups enjoy as they engage in the creative process.

Once group members feel comfortable with the material, the activity can be presented in numerous ways to match the needs, preferences, and experiences of a particular group. For some preadolescents, creating with their eyes closed reduces anxiety and self-consciousness and also facilitates inward focus, but some preteen children may experience greater anxiety with their eyes closed. The therapist is always flexible in suggestions and responsive to the individual needs of group members.

The following is an example of a brief guided imagery that I have used with repeated success with preadolescents. I suggest that "some kids like to do this with their eyes closed and be surprised at what they have made."

> Imagine that you have traveled through time into the future where human life as we know it no longer exists. The world is inhabited by thousands of varieties of animals and creatures, big and small—some look like animals that we know today, and others are like no creature that you have ever seen. If you could be any animal or creature in this new world, what would you be? Think about what you look like and begin to shape your animal/creature. When you feel like your creation is mostly formed, if your eyes are closed, open your eyes and look at it and then finish what it needs. You can use any of the materials in the room to make your creature or create a place for it to rest.

When group members finish, they are encouraged to tell about their creation and give it a name if they choose. Encourage connections among group members and a sense of belonging by linking preadolescents' comments as they share their creations with each other. Based on members' immediate needs and building on group members' descriptions of their creatures, additional suggestions from the therapist can facilitate interpersonal sharing among group members within the safety of the metaphor, such as, "What is your animal/creature good at? What does your animal/creature like to do for fun? What is its least favorite thing to do? If your animal/creature had one wish, what would it be?"

Group Projects Using Clay Animals

Extend the activity by suggesting that group members work together to create environments, such as "create a home for your animal/creatures to live together," "create the ideal school," "create a fantasy trip/vacation," and so on.

Note: The first author (Crane) has used this activity, with some modifications, for more than 20 years with individuals, groups, and families. I am indebted to Dr. Mary Costas for her influence in the creation of the Clay Animal Creature.

For the first time, Isabelle spoke up to share her creation before anyone else. "This is Flutterby. She has really strong and beautiful wings so she can fly way up high and go anywhere she wants to go. But, she can also close her wings and make herself into a tiny ball." The therapist reflected, "So, Flutterby can choose when she wants to show her beautiful wings." Isabelle nodded her head and added, "But she also knows when she needs to hide in her special place from the scary animals in the new world" (pointing to her home that she made for Flutterby and showing us the small ball of clay that she tucked behind the waterfall she created). She finished by describing the elaborate "resting place" that she created for Flutterby. It is amazing the amount of detail that preadolescents take from the guided imagery and spontaneously use in their descriptions! Isabelle had a huge smile on her face as Beatrice and Monique asked her questions about her creation and said how much they liked it. It was obvious that Isabelle's internal experience of creating Flutterby and receiving validating feedback from the other girls had been powerful. Although the therapist was aware that other aspects of her creation she had not shared were meaningful, this was not the time to share those observations in the group.

Because of space constraints, the remaining group members' creations are only briefly described. Beatrice named her very colorful creation "Fishy-Wishy" and described her as part fish, part princess, who had special powers to make wishes come true. Monique, who struggled the most with her creation, quietly shared, "This is MuMu, Ruler of the Sea." She described her creature as ruler of a special kingdom in the deepest part of the ocean that only she knew about, but that she could also fly and live outside of the ocean when she chose. The "something wished for" appeared in each of the girl's creations. Each creature possessed special powers that allowed them control over their "new world."

This experience represented a shift in the group dynamics. The girls seemed to recognize and value the deeper level of sharing that resulted from the experience of witnessing and validating each other's creative process. As a result, there was a felt increase in the level of trust and acceptance among the girls that was evident as they shared their snack before transitioning back to their classrooms.

Ending Phase: Mandala-Collage

This activity combines the medium of collage with the practice of mandala-making and is a favorite for bringing closure to preadolescent groups because of its integrative properties, and because it allows group members to take away a tangible representation of their experience within the group.

The creation of mandalas for spiritual and healing purposes has been practiced for thousands of years across cultures (Malchiodi, 2002). Jung (1973), the first to use the mandala as a therapeutic tool, acknowledged their calming and healing effect on individuals as well as their potential for integration. Young (2001) also suggested that mandalas help individuals gain self-awareness through connection of the unconscious to the conscious. Mandala-making consists of creating an image within a circular space. Malchiodi (2002) describes a process for introducing mandalas that we find helpful in adapting for use with preadolescents. Rogers (1993) suggested that collage helps facilitate a focus on process rather than product and is especially helpful for clients who are inhibited by media such as drawing, which is often associated with artistic ability. Incorporating a variety of collage and art materials into mandala-making provides preadolescents with flexibility in creative self-expression. But, at the same time, combining multiple mediums within the powerful image of the mandala can elicit deep feelings that may be out of group members' awareness. For this reason, we suggest this activity be used in the ending phase of therapy, and even then, with respect for group members' emotional readiness.

Materials Needed

Provide a variety of expressive media, including magazines, assorted craft materials, pastels, crayons, markers, assorted glues, and a hot glue gun. Each group member needs a circle-shaped surface to create a mandala. Provide an assortment of sizes and colored paper for drawing or cutting a circle along with circle templates. Inexpensive white paper plates provide a quick alternative that offers a sturdy surface for gluing.

Case Study

The Mandala-Collage activity was presented in session 14, which was the next to the final session, to allow time for the activity to be continued into the next week if necessary. The therapist knew it was important that the girls' last experience together not be rushed and that they experienced a sense of closure. Equally important, group members needed plenty of time to engage in a creative process that permitted integration of their experience.

The play therapist began the session by again reminding the girls that next week would be their last group meeting and then briefly introduced the Mandala-Collage activity. The therapist showed the group members the premade circles, as well as the materials to create their own circles, and offered the following prompt:

> Inside the circle, you can use any of the materials in the room to express your feelings, thoughts, wishes, or anything you want about yourself. These are only suggestions; there is no right or wrong way to create your mandala. You can use any of the materials that you want. (Malchiodi, 2002)

The girls were deeply immersed in creating their mandalas. Although very few words were spoken, there was a tangible connection and comfort level among group members. When there were 15 minutes remaining, the therapist reminded the girls of the time. As a group, the girls decided they wanted more time to finish the next week. They agreed to work five more minutes, then stop for what had become a very important part of their time together—snack time, a time that was more about sharing with each other than about eating.

The following week, the girls agreed that 15 minutes would be ample time to finish their mandala creations and asked the therapist to let them know when 10 minutes had passed. Within moments the girls were again absorbed in creating their mandalas, and they reluctantly added the finishing touches at the agreed-upon time. Beatrice was typically the most social of the girls, but in this session she was more pensive and had the most difficulty ending. She spent the majority of the time in both mandala sessions on an elaborate and multilayered object in the center of her circle. She was the first to speak after the girls gathered in a circle to share their last creation together. She said that she really liked her mandala, and that this was her favorite activity. She pointed to images around the outside of the circle and stated those represented her friends and included Isabelle, Monique, and the therapist as the largest images. Next, she pointed to the middle that contained a large black felt circle with colorful feathers glued on top. "That represents me when we started group. I wanted everyone to see me as beautiful like my sister, but underneath . . ." Beatrice hesitated a moment, "I knew I wasn't." Then she lifted the felt to allow the others to see the part that was hidden, an iridescent fabric with beads glued to the top. "This shows me on the inside, but I don't usually let anyone see that part." The therapist reflected, "Except maybe in here." Beatrice nodded and smiled. It was clear that she was reflecting on her experience, but she chose not to share more with the group.

Beatrice's sharing at such a deep level seemed to set the tone for the group's last session. Although neither Monique nor Isabelle verbally shared as much, their mandalas were obviously meaningful. Most important, group members' empathy and acceptance as they witnessed each others' creations served as a powerful therapeutic experience, which would not be possible in individual play therapy. The therapist intentionally encouraged group members' expressions of happiness and sadness that were so vividly reflected in their creations. Ending the group was sad, but also a celebration of the fun and closeness they had shared. The girls decided the week before to bring a special treat for their last time together, and as a surprise for the therapist. Their mood was noticeably light while they reminisced about their time together over the past 15 weeks and decorated the holiday cookies for their special surprise. Isabelle had baked the cookies at home, Beatrice brought the icing, and Monique supplied the decorations. This final activity, planned and carried out by the group members, was yet another indication of the sense of belonging and connection that had formed.

This case example briefly illustrates the integration of expressive arts and group play therapy with a preadolescent group of girls. Using a humanistic approach, the play therapist used a balance of therapist-guided expressive art experiences with unstructured play and creative experiences to provide group members with a safe and accepting environment to explore, create, negotiate, and solve their own problems.

CONCLUSION

Through the use of play and expressive media, children symbolically express thoughts and feelings they may be unable to communicate verbally. According to Winnicott (1971), "It is in playing and only in playing that the individual child or adult is able to be creative and to use the whole personality, and it is only in being creative that the individual discovers the self" (p. 54). Integrating play therapy and expressive arts within a humanistic framework provides a developmentally responsive and nonthreatening means for preadolescents to engage in the creative process of self-discovery. The group format offers additional advantages by tapping into preteens' developmental need for a felt sense of belonging outside of their families and by providing a safe environment in which they can explore the self in relation to others and experiment with more satisfying ways of connecting socially. Through this creative process, preadolescents more fully develop their internal resources for self-regulation, self-responsibility, and self-direction, as well as their capacity for satisfying and intimate relationships.

REFERENCES

Akos, P., Hamm, J. V., Mack, S., & Dunaway, M. (2007). Utilizing the developmental influences of peers in middle school groups. *Journal of Specialists in Group Work*, *32*(1), 51–60.

Akos, P., & Martin, M. (2003). Transition groups for preparing students for middle school. *Journal of Specialists in Group Work*, *28*(2), 139–154.

Armstrong, S. (2008). *Sandtray therapy: A humanistic approach*. Dallas, TX: Ludic Press.

Association for Play Therapy. (2013). Retrieved from http://a4pt.com

Badenoch, B. (2008). *Being a brain-wise therapist: A practical guide to interpersonal neurobiology*. New York, NY: W. W. Norton.

Baggerly, J., Ray, D., & Bratton, S. (2010). *Child-centered play therapy research: The evidence base for effective practice*. Hoboken, NJ: Wiley.

Bratton, S., Ceballos, P., & Ferebee, K. (2009). Integration of structured activities within a humanistic group play therapy format for preadolescents. *Journal of Specialists in Group Work, 34*(3), 251–275.

Bratton, S., & Ferebee, K. W. (1999). The use of structured expressive art activities in group activity therapy with preadolescents. In D. S. Sweeney & L. E. Homeyer (Eds.), *The handbook of group play therapy* (pp. 192–214). San Francisco, CA: Jossey-Bass.

Bratton, S., & Ray, D. (2002). Humanistic play therapy. In D. Cain & J. Seeman (Eds.), *Humanistic psychotherapies: Handbook of research and practice* (pp. 369–402). Washington, DC: American Psychological Association.

Bratton, S., Ray, D., Rhine, T., & Jones, L. (2005). The efficacy of play therapy with children: A meta-analytic review of treatment outcomes. *Professional Psychology: Research and Practice, 36*(4), 376–390.

Brown, S. (2009). *Play: How it shapes the brain, opens the imagination, and invigorates the soul.* New York, NY: Penguin.

Center for Play Therapy. (2013). Retrieved from http://cpt.unt.edu/shopping/bibliography.aspx

Chapman, L. (1993). Establishing a pediatric art and play therapy program in a community hospital. In E. Virshup (Ed.), *California art therapy trends* (pp. 219–230). Chicago, IL: Magnolia Street.

Chapman, L. M., Morabito, D., Ladakakos, C., Schreier, H., & Knudson, M. M. (2001). The effectiveness of art therapy interventions in reducing Posttraumatic Stress Disorder (PTSD) symptoms in pediatric trauma patients. *Art Therapy: Journal of the American Art Therapy Association, 18*(2), 100–104.

Davis, S. (2002). Psychological contact through person-centered expressive arts. In G. Wyatt & P. Sanders (Eds.), *Rogers' therapeutic conditions: Evolution, theory, and practice: Contact and perception* (Vol. 4, pp. 204–220). Manchester, UK: PCCS Books.

De Domenico, G. (1999). Group sandtray-worldplay. In D. Sweeney & L. Homeyer (Eds.), *The handbook of group play therapy* (pp. 215–233). San Francisco, CA: Jossey-Bass.

Draper, K., Ritter, K. B., & Willingham, E. U. (2003). Sand tray group counseling with adolescents. *The Journal for Specialists in Group Work, 28*(3), 244–260.

Erikson, E. H. (1980). *Identity and the life cycle.* New York, NY: W. W. Norton.

Favara-Scacco, D., Smirne, G., Schiliro, G., & Di Cataldo, A. (2001). Art therapy as support for children with leukemia during painful procedures. *Medical Pediatric Oncology, 36*(4), 478–480.

Flahive, M. W., & Ray. D (2007). Effect of group sandtray therapy with preadolescents. *The Journal for Specialists in Group Work, 32*(4), 362–382.

Gerrity, D. A., & DeLucia-Waack, J. L. (2007). Effectiveness of groups in the schools. *Journal of Specialists in Group Work, 32*(1), 97–106.

Gil, E. (1991). The *healing power of play: Working with abused children.* New York, NY: Guilford Press.

Gil, E. (2006). *Helping abused and traumatized children: Directive and non-directive approaches.* New York, NY: Guilford Press.

Gil, E. (2010). *Working with children to heal interpersonal trauma: The power of play.* New York, NY: Guilford Press.

Ginott, H. (1961). *Group psychotherapy with children: The theory and practice of play therapy.* New York, NY: McGraw-Hill.

Ginott, H. (1994). *Group psychotherapy with children: The theory and practice of play therapy* (2nd ed.). Northvale, NJ: Jason Aronson.

Hamachek, D. E. (1988). Evaluating self-concept and ego development within Erikson's psychosocial framework: A formulation. *Journal of Counseling and Development, 66*(8), 354–360.

Homeyer, L., & Sweeney, D. (2010). *Sandtray: A practical manual.* Canyon Lake, TX: Lindan Press.

International Expressive Arts Therapy Association. (2013). *What are the expressive arts?* Retrieved from www.ieata.org

Jung, C. (1973). *Mandala symbolism.* Princeton, NJ: Princeton University Press.

Kalff, D. (1971). *Sandplay: Mirror of a child's psyche.* San Franciso, CA: C. G. Jung Institute.

Kapitan, L. (2010). *Introduction to art therapy research.* New York, NY: Routledge.

Kestley, T. (2010). Group sandplay in elementary schools. In A. Drewes, L. Carey, & C. Schaefer (Eds.), *School-based play therapy* (pp. 329–349). Hoboken, NJ: Wiley.

Landgarten, H. (1981). *Clinical art therapy.* New York, NY: Brunner/Matzel.

Landgarten, H. (1987). *Family art psychotherapy: A clinical guide and casebook.* New York, NY: Brunner/Mazel.

Landreth, G. L. (2012). *Play therapy: The art of the relationship* (3rd ed.). New York, NY: Brunner Routledge.

Lowenfeld, M. (1979). *Understanding children's sandplay: Lowenfeld's World Technique.* London, England: George Allen & Urwin.

Lyshak-Stelzer, F., Singer, P., St. John, P., & Chemtob, C. M. (2007). Art therapy for adolescents with Posttraumatic Stress Disorder symptoms: A pilot study. *Art Therapy: Journal of the American Art Therapy Association, 24*(4), 163–169.

Malchiodi, C. A. (2002). *The soul's palette: Drawing on art's transformative powers*. New York, NY: Guilford Press.

Malchiodi, C. A. (2005). *Expressive therapies*. New York, NY: Guilford Press.

Malchiodi, C. A. (2008). *Creative interventions for traumatized children*. New York, NY: Guilford Press.

National Coalition of Creative Arts Therapies Associations [NCCATA], (2013). http://www.nccata.org.

Oaklander, V. (1988). *Windows to our children: A Gestalt therapy approach to our children and adolescents*. Highland, NY: The Center for Gestalt Development.

Oaklander, V. (2007). *Hidden treasures: A map to the child's inner self*. London, England: Karmac Books.

Oesterreich, L. (1995). Ages & stages—nine through eleven-years-olds. In L. Oesterreich, B. Holt, & S. Karas (Eds.), *Iowa family child care handbook [PM 1541]* (pp. 202–204). Ames: Iowa State University Extension.

Ojiambo, D., & Bratton, S. (in press). Effects of group activity play therapy on problem behaviors of preadolescent Ugandan orphans. *Journal for Counseling and Development*.

Packman, J., & Bratton, S. C. (2003). A school-based group play therapy intervention with learning disabled preadolescents exhibiting behavioral problems. *International Journal of Play Therapy*, *12*(2), 7–29.

Panksepp, J. (2004). *Affective Neuroscience*. London, England: Oxford University Press.

Perry, B. D. (2006). Applying principles of neurodevelopment to clinical work with maltreated and traumatized children: The neurosequential model of therapeutics. In N. B. Webb (Ed.), *Working with traumatized youth in child welfare* (pp. 27–52). New York, NY: Guilford Press.

Piaget, J. (1977). *The development of thought: Equilibrium of cognitive structures*. New York, NY: Viking.

Pifalo, T. (2002). Pulling out the thorns: Art therapy with sexually abused children and adolescents. *Art Therapy: Journal of the American Art Therapy Association*, *19*(1), 12–22.

Pifalo, T. (2006). Art therapy with sexually abused children and adolescents: Extended research study. *Art Therapy: Journal of the American Art Therapy Association*, *23*(4), 181–185.

Ray, D. (2011). *Advanced play therapy: Essential conditions, knowledge, and skills for child practice*. New York, NY: Routledge.

Reddy, L., Files-Hall, T., & Schaefer, C.E. (2005). *Empirically based play interventions for children* (2nd ed.). Washington, DC: American Psychological Association.

Rogers, N. (1993). *The creative connection: Expressive arts as healing.* Palo Alto, CA: Science & Behavior Books.

Rubin, J. (1984). *Child art therapy.* New York, NY: Wiley.

Rubin, J. (2005). *Child art therapy: Twenty-fifth anniversary.* Hoboken, NJ: Wiley.

Rubin, J. (2010). *Introduction to art therapy.* New York, NY: Routledge

Schaefer, C. E. (2011). *Foundations of play therapy.* Hoboken, NJ: Wiley.

Schiffer, M. (1952). Permissiveness versus sanction in activity group therapy. *International Journal of Group Psychotherapy, 2,* 225–261.

Shen, Y. (2007). Developmental model using gestalt play versus cognitive-verbal group with Chinese adolescents: Effects on strengths and adjustment enhancement. *The Journal for Specialists in Group Work, 32*(3), 285–305.

Shen, Y., & Armstrong, S. A. (2008). Impact of group sandtray therapy on the self-esteem of young adolescent girls. *The Journal for Specialists in Group Work, 33*(2), 118–137.

Sholt, M., & Gavron, T. (2006). Therapeutic qualities of clay-work in art therapy and psychotherapy: A review. *Art Therapy: Journal of the American Art Therapy Association, 23*(2), 66–72.

Slavson, S. R., & Redl, F. (1944). Levels and applications of group therapy: Some elements in activity group therapy. *American Journal of Orthopsychiatry, 14,* 578–588.

Slavson, S., & Schiffer, M. (1975). *Group psychotherapies for children: A textbook.* New York, NY: International Universities Press.

Smitheman-Brown, V., & Church, R. P. (1996). Mandala drawing: Facilitating creative growth in children with ADD or ADHD. *Art Therapy: Journal of the American Art Therapy Association, 13*(4), 252–262.

Sweeney, D., & Homeyer, L. (1999). Group play therapy. In D. Sweeney & L. Homeyer (Eds.), *Handbook of group play therapy: How to do it, how it works, whom it's best for* (pp. 3–14). San Francisco, CA: Jossey-Bass.

Vygotsky, L. (1966). Play and its role in the mental development of the child. *Vaprosy psikhologi, 12,* 6–18.

Wilson, K., & Ryan, V. (2005). *Play therapy: A non-directive approach for children and adolescents* (2nd ed.). London, England: Bailliere Tindall.

Winnicott, D. (1971). *Playing and reality.* New York, NY: Basic Books.

Young, A. (2001). Mandalas. *Encounter Autumn, 14*(3), 25–34.

Integrating Play and Expressive Art Therapy Into Communities: A Multimodal Approach

JULIA BYERS

INTRODUCTION

The Rabbit Hole has often been referred to as a bizarre or difficult situation in which a nonsensical area of confusion or chaos exists in the midst of real life. Essentially, everything that we believe we know to be true becomes totally out of sync with the reality of what is actually happening. The complex dilemma of what we once knew, trusted, and often took for granted versus what is taking place in reality can cause the normal experience of family and community development to become stunted. Posttraumatic experiences typically occur as a result of violence, natural disasters, or accidents. Single-blow traumatic incidents, like the one used as a case study in this chapter, are yet another subsection of horrible events that can lead to posttraumatic stress disorder (PTSD). How families and a community can climb out of this far-reaching predicament and out of the chaos of the ensuing Rabbit Hole is the focus of this chapter.

For the protection of family members, the location and demographics of the people, town, and school are referred to using pseudonyms. This narrative heuristic inquiry focuses on a crisis intervention that integrates expressive arts with play therapy. Moreover, it reflects on the integrated use of these expressive approaches with elementary schoolchildren, parents, and siblings, and the local school and town communities.

> One ordinary Saturday morning, when 7-year-old Joe invited his best friend Tim over to watch Saturday morning cartoons and play, the unimaginable happened. Joe's trusted and beloved pet dog inadvertently killed Tim when the front door was opened to let Tim inside. Apparently, there had been a ruckus in Tim's family's yard when three dogs had trespassed onto the property and were running around. Joe's family dog, a Rottweiler, had become agitated at the barking and lunged at Tim when he came through the door. The extremely surreal event of the death of the child was witnessed by Joe, Joe's two older siblings, and two neighbors. During the incident, Joe's father was sleeping upstairs while Joe's mother was at the grocery store. The extraordinary complexity of the psychological and emotional responses for Joe, both families who had lived in houses side-by-side since the children's births, neighbors, schoolmates, parents at the school, local citizens, and beyond, represents an irreparable moment in time. There was neither an easy escape nor answer to help the community heal. All were plunged into the Rabbit Hole.

The purpose of this chapter is to illustrate how the integration and use of expressive art/play therapy provided assistance to a community in crisis. This extraordinary experience, found within the normalcy of everyday life, highlights the vulnerability of all growing families and the indescribable, relatively unpredictable nature of being human. Witnessing one's pet kill a person, especially at the age of 7, can be a terrifying experience, compromising a child's sense of safety and stability.

This chapter begins with a brief review of commentary on the 2012 community disaster of Sandy Hook Elementary School, supported by posttraumatic stress literature in mental health communities. Related issues such as children's magical thinking response, underdeveloped sense of the concept of death, absolute need for safety, signs of ongoing distress and their need for expression, cognitive reframing, and mastering of emotions can be assessed through the specific techniques of integrated expressive media. The aim is to help children appropriately or adequately express their thoughts and feelings to reduce long-term psychological deterioration. A brief review of current literature in the expressive art/play therapy field supports the use of this analytic, therapeutic approach to cope with issues in crisis intervention.

The specific family, classroom, school, and community response in the case study of Tim and Joe is described to help demonstrate how elements in the system worked together to support each other. Examples of the brief intervention and follow-up team's response to the disaster are presented. The existential predicament of human responses is highlighted by the opportunities afforded by the expression and play of the arts to provide a form of psychological and emotional expression and eventual resolution.

CONTEXT

I was already familiar with the community and school system in the quaint New England town before this single-blow traumatic incident occurred. I had previously been called in to help the school community cope with an incident involving the former superintendent, who had been found guilty of stealing money from the town and school. The shock of betrayal was differential but still deeply felt by staff members and students, according to their historical relationship with the authority figure. To help the academic and larger community start to manage the situation and their emotions, I developed a relational process of helping the educational leaders find mediating ways of communicating among the six schools. The current superintendent was familiar with my previous work in the school community and my crisis intervention work in the Middle East. She contacted me the Sunday immediately following the single-blow incident to provide an immediate triage of mental health support for the school community and beyond.

During the period in which I was writing this chapter, the horrific event of a gunman killing 20 children and six staff members at Sandy Hook Elementary School in Newtown, Connecticut, occurred. I felt compelled to review the reporting of the media and experts' immediate response to the public within the first week of the tragedy to help readers understand what sort of current methods are being used in single-blow traumatic incidents. Also, the incidents involved with the mass murder at Sandy Hook Elementary have been intertwined throughout this chapter to provide readers with additional contextualization of trauma's impact on both children witnessing it in the community and as clinicians invested in children's mental health within the community.

Although there is a gap in the literature, especially within the expressive therapy field, specifically addressing how to respond to the very specific crisis of a family pet killing a neighbor, there is an increasing body of literature on coping with PTSD and community crisis intervention. Although the violence of an enraged 20-year-old's shooting within the school premises at Sandy Hook rings sadly reminiscent of the Columbine Massacre in Colorado in 1999 and the 2007 shootings at Virginia Tech, the crisis at Sandy Hook was indescribably horrific and distinguishable in the witnessing of violence and deaths by and of elementary-aged schoolchildren. Given the ages (6 to 7 years old) of the immediate friends, and the role of classmates, neighbors, and family within the communities in the case of both Sandy Hook and with Tim and Joe, the implications of how a young child processes these types of incidents needs special consideration.

According to Bynner and Wadsworth (2010), the brain of a 7-year-old child is at a developmental stage in which magical thinking occurs; it is often difficult to distinguish reality from fantasy. From a cognitive perspective, children of this age require an adult or significant caregiver to help them understand that the deceased friend is not in pain or feeling lonely. The concept of the friend never returning needs clarification. As Stephen Brock (as referenced in Arrillaga, 2012) instructs, children instinctively look to adults, whether teachers or family members, to find cues for their overall behavior and responses with others. As Garbarino (as referenced in Neergaard, 2012) and others suggest to parents, caregivers, and teachers who are in contact with children who have witnessed these kinds of trauma, the goal is to foster a sense of security. Last, Carol North emphasizes how important and powerful the support of people who went through the traumatic event together can be (Neergaard, 2012).

Researchers (Adler-Nevo & Manassis, 2005; Ayyash-Abdo, 2001; Chemtob, Nakashima, & Carlson, 2002; Cohen, Mannarino, Greenberg, Padlo, & Shipley, 2002; Cook et al., 2005; Feeny, Foa, Treadwell, & March, 2004; Malchiodi, 2003) found that it is typical for children to experience nightmares, trouble sleeping, and the need to stay close to loved ones, as well as to feel nervous, agitated, jumpy, or moody after witnessing a violent trauma. The vicarious secondary trauma can also cause symptoms of stress for people near to the person who died. When symptoms continue or increase into depression and anxiety for more than a couple of weeks, children often need further professional intervention. Family therapy or group therapy is often advised in follow-up support, depending on how close the relationships are to the grieving family members. As Brock (as cited in Arrillaga, 2012) advises, "Having specific procedures to follow probably helps keep youngsters calm and focused and could potentially minimize the effects of a trauma down the road" (para. 11).

An official Newtown Schools and Town e-mail message from the principal of Sandy Hook Elementary School, distributed through *School Messenger* service (School Messenger is a notification service used by the nation's leading school systems to connect with parents, students, and staff through voice, SMS text, e-mail, and social media) following the tragedy, identified the enemy of healing as "isolation." Her comforting words to the community focused on the fact that isolation can feed fear and anger in all members of the community. The antidote response is to encourage community-compassionate exchanges that include some recognition of good qualities, such as acknowledging and valuing the empathetic care and goodwill of all, to create a sense of safety.

Even children as young as first graders can benefit from cognitive-behavioral therapy in learning to identify and label feelings such as anger, frustration, worry, and how to balance a worried thought with a brave one (Neergaard, 2012). What was evident in the media reports of the events at Sandy Hook was the focus on the younger children's ability to make sense of the trauma through play. As reported by Biel (as referenced in Neergaard, 2012), "Youngsters may pull out action figures or stuffed animals and re-enact what they had witnessed, perhaps multiple times." In this way, 6- and 7-year-old children can gain mastery over their overwhelming feelings associated with the trauma.

Also, the encouragement for children to draw after a horrific experience helps them to organize their thoughts and provide an avenue for adults to assess what they are thinking and feeling and check for distortions in order to keep reality in check. As Elaine Ducharme, a trauma specialist, advised on *National Public Radio* (Simon & Ducharme, 2012), the drawings are truly important to know more about how children are processing their emotions. A 6- or 7-year-old also may not be able to understand the concept of time in a mature sense, such as seeing images of the trauma repeatedly on TV, and feeling or believing the events are reoccurring. If adults are able to get their own emotions in perspective/balance and are able to reassure children that they are safe, there is a higher prognosis of returned normalcy in the everyday lives of witnesses (adapted from Ducharme's interview with Scott Simon on National Public Radio, November 2012, entitled, "To Recover from Trauma, Kids Follow Lead of Adults.")

In reviewing the public media commentary following the horror of the Sandy Hook shooting, it became apparent that understanding the developmental age of children who were affected was extremely important in helping these children to gain mastery over their feelings. The power of community support and a need to have a focused triage plan of intervention to avoid feelings of isolation are paramount, as is the general public awareness and encouragement to utilize play, art, and other expressive media to process multiple levels of coping.

SCHOOL COMMUNITY RESPONSE

As briefly described at the beginning of the chapter, in response to a schoolchild's single-blow trauma of witnessing his beloved dog kill his best friend, the exceptional leadership of this particular town's superintendent was noteworthy. Several hours after the incident occurred, the local fire/emergency department contacted the superintendent to apprise her of the situation. The goal was to initiate an immediate triage for the family, neighbors, and friends of the boys in the town of 10,000 people. Responsible for the six schools in the town, the superintendent immediately focused on the primary elementary school where the boys were both students, first alerting the principal and school counselors of the situation. The superintendent then immediately contacted me to ask of my availability to provide counseling for the community. Within hours, we had set up an emergency room of sorts where neighbors, friends, and parents could come to share their grief and concerns. Because the local school counselors were employed in permanent positions, the administrative team of 12 personnel and outside consultants encouraged specific counselors to be available for the families of both Tim and Joe. Because neighbors had witnessed the event and still others saw the fire trucks, ambulances, and other emergency vehicles rush down the street, the triage center at the school became an important venue for them to express their multitude of emotional concerns.

We also organized and announced a parents' evening to take place two days later to answer questions and concerns focusing on the psychoeducation of the complicated grieving process, and to reduce the corresponding fears accompanying the parents' own responses. John Woodall, school staff, and I fielded questions such as, "What do I tell my children about what happened?" and, "How do we help them feel safe with their own pets?" Yet others focused on investigating stricter laws and provisions addressing the supervision of dogs, the use of leashes, and so on. Subsequently, ongoing follow-up group counseling sessions were made available for the parents.

For my part in the rapid intervention, I instituted expressive therapy at the elementary school for the general public and two sessions of follow-up treatment in the 7-year-old boys' classroom to assess whether certain children experienced PTSD symptoms beyond the normal grieving response. Two weeks after the single-blow traumatic incident, I went with three graduate students into Tim's first-grade homeroom to facilitate an informal assessment. Out of approximately 20 students, only three were identified as exhibiting psychological maladjusted symptoms beyond the normal range.

SHATTERED WORLDVIEW

The expectation that home should represent a place that provides a sense of safety, protection, love, and nurturing warmth is the hope of all families. As in the Greek word *thémi*, meaning "what is right," the loss of a trustworthy structure such as home can have catastrophic results if all the rules a family ever lived by are broken. The trust falters if parents cannot protect, or if a beloved family dog attacks; the sense of safety is betrayed, and a growing child feels guilt and shame about being unable either to rescue his friend or control his dog. This rips at the fabric or foundation of our *thémis*, creating an existential crisis that is much more complicated than sudden death through illness or accident. When Joe and others witnessed the violence of the family Rottweiler unleashed on 45-pound Tim, they encountered an aberrant, horrific event. Exposure to complex trauma can result in a loss of the ability to maintain interpersonal relatedness and challenge the child with lifelong problems of self-regulation. Resulting impairments include psychiatric and addictive disorders, chronic medical illness, and legal, vocational, and familial problems (Cook et al., 2005).

Accepting the reality of the loss of a child and the death of the dog through euthanasia deeply affected both families, who had lived side by side harmoniously as their children were growing up. The fact that Tim's mother, who happened to be a nurse, was unable to resuscitate her child after the other children ran to her for help, or the fact that Joe's father could not get the dog to loosen its death grip on Tim, exacerbated feelings of helplessness and guilt. There was also the stigma and blame by the community of Joe's family for owning a Rottweiler dog, a breed publically recognized for its aggressive, protective, and guarding behaviors. The dark side of humanity was exposed. As Yeats (1919) captures in his poem, "The Second Coming":

> Things fall apart; the centre cannot hold;
> Mere anarchy is loosed upon the world,
> The blood-dimmed tide is loosed, and everywhere
> The ceremony of innocence is drowned;
> The best lack all conviction, while the worst
> Are full of passionate intensity.

As documented by Gil (2006, 2010, 2012), Malchiodi (2008), and Rubin (2001, 2005), the use of both play and art therapy (the imaginative realm of symbols and image making), with the additional use of expressive media such as music, movement, and drama, can provide children and their families and friends with a creative avenue for exploring their worries and psychological suffering induced by traumatic events. Malchiodi (2003) suggested the use of a Magic Book or My Safe Box as vehicles for children to cope with their anxiety and master a sense of control when all things feel and are, quite frankly, in chaos in the immediate aftermath of a trauma. Under normal circumstances, grief is most often experienced as intense, and in single-blow traumatic incidents that result in death, it is only more intensified.

The Magic Book encourages children to problem solve and find answers to the burdening questions they might have. The therapist prompts the child to image a Magic Book that will serve as a good listener and provide feedback. Through drawing representations of worries or fears, and by adding colors and textures, the projected book adds important chapters to the child's life. The Safe Box can be a shoebox or any handmade or found container. The child is encouraged to gather and collect in the box a variety of photographs and objects that are special in memory of a loved one. This Safe Box provides a safe place, helping a child to feel at ease during the most stressful times, including times of separation and loss.

The complexity of the issues can be witnessed in the metaphoric communication seen when the integration of expressive arts/play therapy is employed. In the integration of therapeutic counseling and the actual interplay of expressive therapies, I have found that the play of the action-oriented modalities serves as the mediator in the understanding of the range of emotions that arise. As in the Axline (1969) and Moustakas (1973) approach to therapy, I tend to employ a more nondirective approach in the immediacy of a rapid response team in order to assess a child's innate coping skills and strengths. I look for the tendency of a particular child to exhibit PTSD after the expected two- to three-week period of shock and work-through. It is more common to use a directive approach, initiating questions such as, "What worries you?" (Malchiodi, 2003), or to encourage a narrative retelling of the trauma. For instance, the therapists might ask the child, "Worry looks like what?" or whatever the child finds frightening since the occurrence of the tragedy and have them draw it out or depict it artistically.

Children and families experience grief differently and uniquely (Green & Connolly, 2009). Some tend to feel numb or to avoid, shut down, and isolate themselves from others, whereas others feel compelled to reenact or retell the horror of the situation in order to make some meaning or sense out of the irrational situation.

Even children who have not directly witnessed the loss of life, but are classmates or friends of those who have, can have severe reactions that are permeated with fear of what could or may happen to them. In my experience, children's imaginations can easily distort the actual, pragmatic environmental angst. To reduce the pressure children might feel to talk or to "do well" during a session (particularly within a school setting, or if parents protectively brought their child in to be checked for unusual behaviors), the act of *being* through the play between words and arts expression is particularly well-suited to children's diverse developmental needs. Similarly, the encouragement of giving assigned children a way to exchange and engage in each others' productions and the process of expression through the arts becomes a metaphoric safe ground away from the bustle of adults, who may be revealing their own worries, questions, and fears.

Although the main goal is to help significant adults relate to their children in long-lasting, helpful ways, in the case of single-blow traumatic incidents, adults often need to seek their own therapeutic resources to enable them to prepare for helping their children. Analogous to grabbing the oxygen masks in an airplane crash, in order to be more present and able to help their children, parents are instructed to put their own masks on before helping their children. The necessity to provide rapid relief opportunities for the children and/or family groups as well as adult counseling is even more paramount. The ability of community members to be present for and supportive of each other is the hallmark of successful responses to community disasters.

EXPRESSIVE THERAPIES HAVEN

Far from a real haven and more in the imaginary sense, a conference room at the primary school was chosen as the setting for a mental health triage for parents and children who were deeply affected by the trauma.

As the local school counselors provided assistance to the immediate family members of those involved in the tragic event, I was available for the neighbors and friends to receive some respite from the crisis. Having little time to gather supplies and knowing that the school had only basic art supplies of crayons, markers, paint, paper, glue, and so on, I grabbed my portable miniature toys, which are commonly used in the technique of sandtray therapy (Homeyer, 2011).

There are several ways to engage children in expressive media. In my experience with crisis intervention work (Byers, 2011), I use what is in the local environment and integrate the use of play and art materials to illuminate the metaphoric value of the individual communication tools. For instance, the use of string, wire, rubber bands, wool, and so forth are literal connectors from one object to another. The emotional significance of the need to attach can be seen in the tension of knots, overbinding, stretch, and flexibility of the chosen material. Also, the movement and placement of fabrics and other representations of boundaries or open drawn spaces can reveal a child's need to encompass, or envelop, another object as guarded protections from another or, alternatively, to self-regulate emotional outbursts that would be directed toward others.

Because the children I was working with generally felt betrayed with a lost sense of trust and safety, I provided large sheets of blank paper or cardboard as a foundation on which they could encounter and engage in different forms of expression. I encouraged them to deploy the miniature toys, which were given to them in thematic clusters: animals, vehicles, scenery (trees, fences, ponds, etc.), people, superheroes, monsters, war toys, and so on. In another canvas bag, I also brought percussion instruments, drums, shaky beans, and small string harmonic instruments, and a variety of colored silk scarves, peacock feathers, balls, and other movement objects. Because of the small space and the timing of the intervention when the community was still in shock, the animated use of more action-oriented large interactions was not used nor truly available.

Although I saw about 20 people seeking immediate counseling, for the purpose of this chapter, I will comment only on three children who represent the range of emotions expressed in the following sections.

Concept of Death

Don, another 7-year-old friend of Tim and Joe's, witnessed the actual incident at Joe's home. Don had been watching the TV in the den when the startling noises of the dog growling and Tim's terrified shouts prompted Don to see what was going on. Don heard Joe's terrified screams for his dad while trying to get the dog away from his best friend. When Don's father heard the sirens of the police and other emergency vehicles arrive, he quickly ran to see what he could do to help. Seeing the commotion of other neighborhood children standing outside watching, Don's father quickly brought his son and the other children to his home for sanctuary. The next day, upon hearing about the intervention, he brought the children to the school.

Don was quick to pick up the animal toys, frantically gathering them in his hands and then letting them drop or crash onto his cardboard foundation. Don's pressured talk focused on the blood "that touched everything and everyone" (Figure 12.1). He drew quick darts of blood on the paws of the creatures and repeatedly demonstrated how "blood was everywhere." In his retelling, the dog also was bleeding from the bystanders' attempts to release Tim. Don stated that he just knew something bad was going to happen that day. The three friends had been playing together but ended up fighting over whose turn it was to play a game. Don just knew it was a bad sign. As Don displayed going in and out of reality between the actual traumatic event and talking about wild animals attacking each other, he muttered that he wondered if "Tim was in pain." He knew he had died, but he just was not sure where exactly he had gone. His father had told Don that Tim was never coming back, but Don wondered if Tim would feel lonely without his friends, and he vowed that they would play well if Tim decided to return. *SpongeBob Square Pants* was on the TV that fateful Saturday morning. Don wondered aloud what SpongeBob would think.

Battles

Zack, a neighbor and classmate on the street, did not witness the event but heard the commotion on the street and learned of the event from what he heard his parents discussing at dinnertime. Zack took the Craypas (oil pastels/crayons) and started making a large field with fences

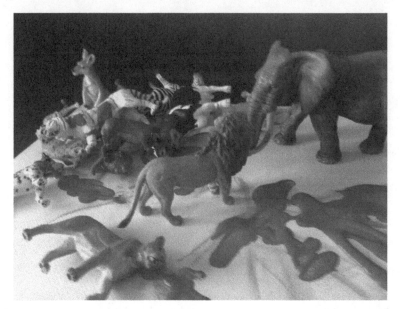

Figure 12.1 Don's Tray

denoting the boundaries of a battlefield. Zack lined up the army soldiers and put cowboys on the opposing side. He then repeatedly reenacted a battle between the fighting units, complete with smashing and take-over yells. He remained focused on the good and evil aspects of the fight, waiting for the superhero to arrive to put an end to the fight. The super-hero, which was off to the side, never came—the battle would not end.

Lack of Protection

Yvonne, a 10-year-old neighbor and friend of Joe's sister, had also wit-nessed the single-blow traumatic incident. A young girl with an apparently relatively loud personality, Yvonne had remained distant and withdrawn for the 24 hours following the incident. She was afraid to tell anyone that she thought it was her dog that had trespassed onto Joe's family's back-yard and started the trouble that caused Joe's dog to act aggressively at the front door. She had heard Joe's dog barking at other dogs in the backyard but kept on watching the TV, assuming that other family members would attend to the disruption. When the violence occurred, Yvonne felt frozen in fear, unable to move or say anything. In retrospect, she blamed herself for not speaking up, which in her mind would have saved Tim's life.

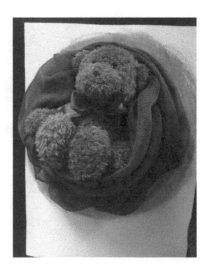

Figure 12.2   Yvonne's "Cold" Teddy Bear

During our time together, Yvonne fidgeted with the ear of a soft teddy bear and repeatedly wrapped the bear in scarves and materials, layering the toy "because it was cold" (Figure 12.2). At home, Yvonne was now afraid to let her dog into her bedroom and reportedly ran into different rooms when her dog appeared. Yvonne did not know if she would ever be able to forgive her dog for causing the trouble that ended in Tim's death. Her parents had reported that they doubted that their dog had trespassed, because it was always on a leash outside. Yvonne was able to draw her teddy bear surrounded by thick walls, denoting a safe place. She imagined how horrible Tim's parents must feel in losing their son. She did not know how to help them, considering it was "her fault" that her dog had gone where he was not supposed to go.

Cognitive Reframing

Integrating expressive arts and play materials afforded these children with an outlet to communicate their fears, worries, and distortions about the single-blow traumatic incident. Through the nondirective invitations to use any and all expressive materials, the nonjudgmental setting, and the expectation that going to the school would be helpful to the children, Don, Zack, and Yvonne used the time to witness each other's responses, gain gentle adult guidance, and to become educated about other children's range of normal feelings and feel in a safe environment in which they could be heard. Each child was recommended for follow-up counseling and support, and the parents were given grief psychoedu-cational information on what to expect within the next two weeks. The parents were also encouraged to attend the parents' psychoeducational information session that evening to address each other's concerns and to offer support and assistance to other parents.

Honoring

Two weeks later, I took three graduate students with me to conduct a session in the classroom of the deceased boy. When we first entered the first-grade classroom, I was struck by how many teddy bears and other stuffed animals sat on or beside each child's desk. Even more apparent was the fact that many children actually had their transitional objects (Winnicott, 2005) in their arms or on their laps. Initially, we gathered all of the children in a circle to play a gesture game, introducing each other and their playmate objects. Out of 19 children, 2 children had difficulty maintaining eye contact and spontaneously interrupted the flow of the game. The children generally appeared too agitated for con-tinued large group activities, so we asked the children to individually draw how they felt that day. Approximately five children drew some-thing that could be related to the loss of their classmate, while others focused on their breakfast, getting to school, TV shows they watched, and flowers or cars—often gender-related items. We broke into four groups in order to witness and acknowledge the children's expression more closely.

As advised by the counselors and myself, the teacher had already begun a book to honor Tim's life. All of the children were given a page on which to draw something they remembered about their classmate that they wanted to give to the grieving family. Because Tim's desk would be removed on the Monday after the upcoming weekend, the children made a collective poem/song about Tim. This activity marked the end of leaving Tim's desk as an icon of saying good-bye. One of the girls who had a difficult time in the opening group brought up the fact that Joe's dog was also in heaven. This raised a flurry of responses by the classmates, either expressing sympathy for or rage at the dog. The children had been informed that it was an accident and that bad things sometimes happen. If they were worried, they were told to talk with their parents or to participate that day in a special time with visitors who cared about the school and the community. In a ritualized fashion, we collectively completed the book for Tim's family.

In the second session a week later, we invited the children to get into the same small groups as the previous week and to build together a puppet show on the theme, "If I Were King/Queen for a Day." The objective was to witness any psychological residue of the single-blow traumatic incident that needed further clarity, or if any children were still experiencing traumatic symptomatology. The theme of mastery and control was displayed by the children and provided a glimpse at how they were returning to normalcy through community support. The power of supportive adults, teachers, friends, and so on, who let the children know that they are truly there for them, is an invaluable gift for life. We ended our session with the kids by sharing the shows and bearing witness to the struggles they were still facing with Tim's death.

The Rabbit Hole

During the trial of "Who Stole the Tarts" in Lewis Carroll's adapted *Alice in Wonderland* (2010), a poem of evidence is read to the court by the White Rabbit:

> They told me you had been to her,
> And mentioned me to him:
> She gave me a good character,
> But said I could not swim.

> He sent them word I had not gone
> (We know it to be true):
> If she should push the matter on,
> What would become of you?

> I gave her one, they gave him two,
> You gave us three or more;
> They all returned from him to you,
> Though they were mine before.

If I or she should chance to be
Involved in this affair,
He trusts to you to set them free,
Exactly as we were.

My notion was that you had been
(Before she had this fit)
An obstacle that came between
Him, and ourselves, and it.

Don't let him know she liked them best,
For this must ever be
A secret, kept from all the rest,
Between yourself and me. (pp. 169–170)

After hearing this evidence, Alice looks around the court and asks, "Is there *anyone* who can explain those verses? . . . I don't believe there's *any* meaning in it" (p. 171). Throughout Carroll's story, Alice is the only one who makes any sense in the tale of nonsense. Single-blow traumatic incidents experienced at the age of 6 or 7, with the complex dynamics of all parties involved, require confronting the random senselessness of life itself, just as Alice, the universal symbol of the individualized child, had to confront the senselessness of the Rabbit Hole in order to get out. Trying to blame and being overwhelmed by feelings of anger, fear, guilt, or dismay can dictate a long road to finding the survivor's feelings of joy, love, and forgiveness. From my experience as a crisis interventionist, there is no one way a parent, a teacher, or a child finds acceptance of horrible loss. However, the expression of integrating the multiple senses through the expressive arts constitutive of our humanity allows opportunities for psychological healing. The epilogue of this crisis is that the strength of the community was profound in supporting the choice of the families not to sue each other, the choice of the school community not to divide over shoulds or should nots, and the effort of the counselors to offer ongoing follow-up for Joe and his family.

As discussed in the beginning of this chapter, children often look to adults for guidance, especially in times of trauma and chaos. A compassionate response generally leads to a higher prognosis of appropriate readaptation to life. The complexity of emotions is often difficult to untangle, but the ability of human service professionals to give aesthetic and emotional distancing through the expressive arts media before children are able or willing to express their concerns in words can help untangle those emotions. As integrative expressive art therapists, we strive to use the spontaneity of the moment to increase communication. Having actual or created objects—ones even as simple as Kleenex tissue—nearby to hold, discard, crush, or twist, provides another avenue to work with understanding. Survivors' guilt for many who witnessed the Sandy Hook shootings or the violence of a beloved pet killing a friend in one's home can be buried and expressed as posttraumatic symptomatology. Integrating play and expressive art therapy ultimately focuses on the full psychological integration of unresolved feelings beyond the catharsis of expression for the child, community, and beyond.

REFERENCES

Adler-Nevo, G., & Manassis, K. (2005). Psychosocial treatment of pediatric traumatic stress disorder: The neglected field of single-incident trauma. *Depression and Anxiety, 22,* 177–189.

Arrillaga, P. (2012, December 19). How prepared can we be if evil strikes again? *The Associated Press.* Retrieved from http://bigstory.ap.org/article/how-prepared-can-we-be-if-evil-strikes-again

Axline, V. (1969). *Play therapy.* New York, NY: Ballantine Books.

Ayyash-Abdo, H. (2001). Childhood bereavement: What school psychologists need to know. *School Psychology International, 22,* 417–433. Doi: 10.1177/0143034301224003

Byers, J. (2011). *Humanitarian art therapy and mental health counseling.* Retrieved from http://counselingoutfitters.com/ vistas/vistas11/Article_50.pdf

Bynner, J. & Wadsworth, M. (2010). Cognitive capital: The case for a construct. *Logitudinal and Life Course Studies: International Journal, 1*(3), 297–304.

Carroll, L. (2010). *Alice's adventures in wonderland.* Franklin, TN: Dalmatian.

Chemtob, C., Nakashima, J., & Carlson, J. (2002). Brief treatment for elementary school children with disaster-related posttraumatic stress disorder: A field study. *Journal of Clinical Psychology, 58*(1), 99–112.

Cohen, J., Mannarino, A., Greenberg, T., Padlo, S., & Shipley, C. (2002). Childhood traumatic grief: Concepts and controversies. *Trauma, Violence, & Abuse, 3*(4), 307–327. Doi: 10.1177/1524838002237332

Cook, A., Spinazzola, J., Ford, J., Lanktree, C., Blaustein, M., Cloitre, M., . . . van der Kolk, B. (2005). Complex trauma in children and adolescents. *Psychiatric Annals, 35*(5), 390–398.

Feeny, N., Foa, E., Treadwell, K., & March, J. (2004). Traumatic stress disorder in youth: A critical review of the cognitive and behavioral treatment outcome literature. *Professional Psychology: Research and Practice, 35*(5), 466–476.

Gil, E. (2006). *Helping abused and traumatized children: Integrating directive and nondirective approaches.* New York, NY: Guilford Press.

Gil, E. (2010). *Working with children to heal interpersonal trauma: The power of play.* New York, NY: Guilford Press.

Gil, E. (2012). Trauma-focused integrated play therapy (TF-IPT). In P. Goodyear-Brown (Ed.), *Handbook of child sexual abuse: Identification, assessment, and treatment* (pp. 251–278). Hoboken, NJ: Wiley.

Green, E. J., & Connolly, M. (2009). Jungian family sandplay with bereaved children: Implications for play therapists. *International Journal of Play Therapy, 18*(2), 84–98.

Homeyer, L. (2011). *Sand tray therapy: A practical manual* (2nd ed.). New York, NY: Routledge.

Malchiodi, C. (2003). Using creative activities as intervention for grieving children. *Trauma and Loss: Research and Interventions, 3*(1), 34–41.

Malchiodi, C. A. (2008). *Creative interventions with traumatized children.* New York, NY: Guilford Press.

Moustakas, C. (1973). *Children in play therapy.* New York, NY: Jason Aronson.

Neergaard, L. (2012, December 18). Experts: Kids are resilient in coping with trauma. *The Associated Press.* Retrieved from http://www.npr.org/templates/story/story.php?storyId=167563280

Rubin, J. (Ed.). (2001). *Approaches to art therapy:Theory and technique* (3rd ed.). Philadelphia, PA: Brunner-Routledge.

Rubin, J. (2005). *Child art therapy.* Hoboken, NJ: Wiley.

Simon, S. (interviewer), & Ducharme, D. (interviewee). (2012). *To recover from trauma, kids follow lead of adults* [Interview transcript]. Retrieved from National Public Radio's Weekend Edition: www.npr .org/2012/12/15/167321218/to-recover-from-trauma-kids-follow-lead-of-adults

Winnicott, D. (2005). *Playing and reality.* Oxon, UK: Routledge.

Yeats, W. B. (1919). "The Second Coming." In H. Gardner (Ed.), *The new Oxford book of English verse* (pp. 820–821). Suffolk, UK: Oxford University Press.

Author Index

Subject Index